Medicine in Translation

For Naava, Noah, and Ariel

Medicine in Translation

∾ Journeys with My Patients ∾

Danielle Ofri

Beacon Press, Boston

Beacon Press
25 Beacon Street
Boston, Massachusetts 02108-2892
www.beacon.org

Beacon Press books
are published under the auspices of
the Unitarian Universalist Association of Congregations.

13 12 11 10   8 7 6 5 4 3 2 1

This book is printed on acid-free paper that meets the uncoated paper ANSI/NISO
specifications for permanence as revised in 1992.

Text composition by Wilsted & Taylor Publishing Services, Oakland, CA

Library of Congress Cataloging-in-Publication Data

Ofri, Danielle.
Medicine in translation : journeys with my patients / by Danielle Ofri.
p. ; cm.
ISBN 978-0-8070-7320-9 (hardcover : alk. paper)
1. Ofri, Danielle. 2. Physicians—New York (State)—New York—Biography.
3. Immigrants—Medical care—New York (State)—New York.
4. Bellevue Hospital. I. Title.
[DNLM: 1. Ofri, Danielle. 2. Emigrants and Immigrants—New York City—
Personal Narratives. 3. Health Services Accessibility—New York City—
Personal Narratives. WA 300 AN7 O33m 2009]

R154.O37A3 2009
610.92'2—dc22
[B]   2009019977

Part One

ᨆ Chapter One ᨆ

There was a sharp rap at the apartment door. When Samuel Chuks Nwanko opened it, he saw a young man standing in the hallway wearing a stained denim jacket over a University of Nigeria T-shirt. Though he was standing still, his arms and legs were in constant motion, like a jittery insect hovering by a streetlamp. The whites of his eyes were spidered with crimson streaks. He was probably a fellow university student but not in the civil engineering department. Samuel didn't recognize him.

"Are you Chuks?" the student asked, his voice quavering as his Adam's apple bobbed unsteadily.

Probably drunk or high, Samuel thought. Not someone he wanted to let in. His fiancée Alaba and her friend were watching a movie in the bedroom, and he didn't want some stoned student making trouble. Besides, they were about to leave for church and he didn't want to be late. But rudeness would only exacerbate things. "Chuks just left," Samuel said, figuring it wouldn't take much to outsmart a drunk.

The student laughed a thin, drawn-out laugh, reaching toward the door frame for support and stumbling closer to Samuel. His breath was rancid.

Definitely drunk, Samuel thought. Probably brewed his own *ogogoro*. Samuel started inventing another polite excuse to send the student off, but then, out of the corner of his eye, he noticed movement at the end of the hall. Six other students turned the corner, their bodies edging out the light from the weak hallway bulb. As they strode toward his apartment, Samuel realized he was about to be mugged. That was when the student in front of him pulled a homemade gun out of his jacket.

Samuel slammed the front door of the apartment, yanking the lock closed. He threw himself into the bedroom where the movie was playing and locked that door too. Alaba and her friend jumped up from the bed at the sudden noise. Samuel grabbed his cell phone, punched in the number of the police, and started some quick mental calculations: It would probably take five to ten minutes for those guys to break down two wooden doors with locks. The police—if he managed to get through to an officer who wasn't taking a cigarette break and who didn't demand an up-front bribe—might take thirty minutes to arrive. Alaba and her friend could hide themselves under the bed. Samuel would probably have time to throw his laptop under the bed with them, but the TV was a goner for sure. His cash was hidden behind the bureau, but there were seven guys and they'd probably trash the place. The bedroom window was narrow—not practical for escape. In any case, Nigerian building codes didn't provide for fire escapes, so the only option from the fourth floor was a leap to the ground.

But Samuel wasn't even able to complete his thoughts. Within thirty seconds both doors were breached and seven sweating men burst into the bedroom, the gun held aloft like a banner. There was a strange moment of calm, of heaving silence. Every muscle of every person in the room seemed frozen. There was no movement save the nervous darting of twenty eyes sizing up the situation. Samuel's cell phone was still pressed against his ear—his call hadn't even gone through yet.

Then one of the students drew a knife. The blade shimmered as it moved swiftly to knock the phone down.

But what an odd thing to see your own ear topple to the ground yet not feel a thing. Samuel stood staring at the piece of flesh on the ground, unable to react. Rose-like specks of blood bloomed on the edges, strangely alluring and fantastic. He was vaguely aware of Alaba and her friend being hustled out the door, but the air around him had solidified like slate, his body ossified into stone. When the first blow arrived, it was a shattering explosion, pain chiseling in all directions. The gang then pounced—pummeling him with fists, kicking him in the gut, slamming him in the face. His body seemed to dissolve, disconnecting from him, his flesh jellying into nothingness.

They argued over who got to kick where. There didn't seem to be a leader, and they bickered with one another as much as they beat up Samuel. Then there was a silver object that Samuel couldn't identify. It whistled as it raced through the air again and again. It made a distinctive metallic slap each time it contacted his skin. But by then he could feel nothing.

After ten minutes, or maybe fifteen, or maybe thirty, they ceased. Like a communal exhalation, their breath was spent. Samuel lay motionless in the stunned silence, aware that he possessed no sense of his body. He was surprised that thoughts continued to be generated in his head—by all accounts, he should have been unconscious. Perhaps that would be coming soon. He hoped they would begin ransacking his room—that would at least offer a respite. The students stood silently, panting, regrouping. Then one pulled out a five-liter canister.

Water, Samuel thought. He knew of this routine—after the beating, thieves would give the victim water to help him recover just a bit, just enough to reveal where the money and valuables were hidden. Perhaps after he drank some water Samuel would be able to concentrate on memorizing their faces—right now they were a blur. Alaba had probably called the police. It wouldn't matter though—these thieves knew how to be quick. They could dismantle an entire apartment in minutes. By this point, Samuel didn't care. They could take his TV, his laptop, his telephone. He just hoped they wouldn't steal his Bible. It was a gift from his father before he'd left for university. It sat on the bureau, dangerously obvious with its cover of fine mahogany leather.

When Samuel saw the water, a thirst like he'd never experienced before arose in his body. It was like flames engulfing dry tinder. It lapped over his wounds—a sensation of dryness, of evisceration. Even if the water was just to make him talk, he desired it desperately. He would have grabbed the water from their hands if he'd been able.

They held Samuel's mouth open and poured the water in. Samuel waited for the fire to be slaked. He waited for the thirst to be quenched. But nothing registered. He could neither feel nor taste the water. He couldn't even sense that liquid was entering his mouth. But he could see them pouring. He could see the clear liquid streaming from the canister.

Perhaps the fire in him was causing the water to evaporate before it reached his lips. Perhaps his throat had closed up and was refusing water. Perhaps God was testing him, denying him water until his soul was pure enough. Perhaps he was hallucinating and there was no water there at all.

Then Samuel noticed something peculiar. After all the sloppiness of their punches and kicks, the thugs were unusually assiduous in handling the water. If a few drops spilled onto their hands, they spat curses, snapping at one another as they scrambled to wipe it off. That was when it dawned on Samuel that the liquid probably wasn't water. He didn't know what it was because he could feel nothing, but instinct told him to close his mouth and refuse to drink. The attackers grew livid, wrenching his mouth open, dumping the rest of it down his throat. Rivulets sloshed over his face and head.

Then they grabbed a four-by-four plank. With one resonant slam on the head, Samuel was out cold.

The attackers dashed out of the room, leaving the canister of sulfuric acid on the concrete floor.

As was the practice after a student was murdered, classmates printed T-shirts and distributed them as a memorial. SAMUEL CHUKS NWANKO—the legend read under his color photo—4/1/80–2/17/05. One more death attributed to a violent, rapacious society.

Chapter Two

The patient's name appeared African. From his date of birth, I could tell that he was twenty-seven years old. That's all I knew, and when I went out to the waiting room, I scanned for a young, black African male. I was at first puzzled by the person who answered to the name. I couldn't tell if he was black or white—not that it mattered, but names were often mixed up in the waiting room and I needed to be sure he was the correct patient. His face was a patchwork of pink, white, and black. Something about his features didn't make sense, but it was hard to judge, as he wore oversize wraparound silver reflective sunglasses and a fedora hat whose brim rested on the top edge of the sunglasses. His jacket was pulled close around him, and the collar raised high.

I greeted him and shook his hand after confirming his name. I supposed he looked at me, but because of his opaque glasses, I couldn't make eye contact with him. Did he have an ophthalmologic illness? Was he deliberately trying to keep me at a distance? Was this a fashion statement?

"English? French?" I asked as I ushered him into my room.

"Either one," he replied.

Sitting down, he removed neither his hat, nor his coat, nor his glasses. Now that we were sitting only three feet apart, I could see that his face was puckered with stiff ridges and deep gouges, like a hastily pulled wax sculpture. In the center there was no nose, only two nostrils opening up from the rubbery scars of his face. The fibrous lips moved stiffly, and his words were difficult to discern.

"What can I help you with today?" I asked, steeling myself for whatever I might be about to hear.

He pulled a folder from his bag. "I am trying to find out about career training," he said, opening the folder and extracting a sheaf of papers. "I was a civil engineering student and I wish to reenter university to complete my studies. I have been waiting many months for this appointment and I was told that you would be able to help me."

He pressed the papers toward me. They were transcripts from the University of Nigeria, carefully collated and neatly clipped.

I never knew what to expect on Monday afternoons at Bellevue Hospital, because it could run the gamut from the ordinary to the farthest and darkest reaches of the human imagination—though this was the first time someone had come to me for career training advice. Every Monday at one was my slot for a new patient from the Survivors of Torture program.

The Bellevue/NYU Program for Survivors of Torture was started in 1995 by one of my colleagues, Dr. Allen Keller. It seemed a natural development in a place like Bellevue, the largest public hospital in New York City and the oldest in America. Immigrants had always come to Bellevue, but in the 1980s and 1990s—when I did my medical training at Bellevue—there was a sharp increase in the number of patients who needed political asylum.

It was hard to be wholeheartedly happy about the growth and success of the SOT program, as it was commonly called. Despite the depressing fact of the increasing need for its services, the program was a thriving, optimistic organization. Several of the faculty members in the medical clinic at Bellevue volunteered to do the medical evaluations, but most of us limited these to one or two slots per week. Any more than that could be overwhelming.

"I think there might be a slight misunderstanding," I said. "I'm a medical doctor, and this is a general medical clinic. For things like career training and college issues, I think you'd need to talk to the social worker."

There was no way to read Samuel Nwanko's expression, but his taut voice seemed to grow tighter. "I was told that you would be able to help me. I have waited many months for this visit. I need to matriculate back to university."

"I'm so sorry," I said, "but I honestly can't help you with that. I can make sure you get to talk to the social worker, but I can only help with the medical issues."

He leaned back in his chair, increasing the distance between us. "I have waited so long for this visit," he repeated, the anger vivid in his constricted voice.

I usually started my medical histories by asking the patient if she or he had any medical conditions. But such a question, designed to be neutral and free of assumptions, seemed crudely insincere, almost vicious, in view of such obvious facial injuries. But how to ask tactfully?

"I'm sorry if there was any miscommunication about this visit," I said, more than annoyed that someone had given this patient unrealistic expectations, "and I apologize for the long delay in getting the appointment. If there are any medical concerns that you'd like to address, I can try to help you with those."

He nodded slightly, his dissatisfaction palpable. "I have holes in my retinas and I need surgery, but I was told that the only surgeons who can do that are in Boston."

Another brick wall. I doubted that Bellevue had such surgeons, and I was sure I would disappoint him again. "The best I can do here," I said, "is get you an appointment with our ophthalmology clinic and they can help you get to the appropriate specialist."

"I've already seen eye doctors," he said, as sharply as he was able. "I know what I need. I can't wait another three months just to see a regular eye doctor."

The silver reflective sunglasses seemed menacing, but of course they were merely neutral plates of plastic. Without eye contact, and with no facial expression visible on his scarred face, I had no nonverbal cues to help our connection. Given what had transpired so far, this visit seemed doomed to fail.

With SOT patients, it was always difficult for me to ask directly, "What happened?" By the time patients got to me for their medical evaluations, they'd told their stories repeatedly, and I never knew whether they wanted to delve again into their horrors. I always approached this moment with trepidation.

"Would you like to tell me what happened?" I asked. "You don't have to if you don't want to, but it might help me to better understand how I can help you."

I focused on my keyboard as I took notes, concentrating to keep my fingers from slipping off.

Growing up as a pastor's son was not easy. Expectations for behavior, dress, activities were high, and choices nonexistent. Every aspect of Samuel Nwanko's daily existence was determined by his father's involvement in the Pentecostal Church. Samuel's musical talents were corralled into the church choir. His friends were limited to the families his father deemed appropriate. When the time came for Samuel to go to college, Rev. Nwanko chose civil engineering for his son, and he enrolled Samuel in a school six hours south, in Rivers State.

Samuel never felt at ease in his life, even though he was genuinely and deeply religious. The concept of questioning one's parents simply did not exist, so his discomfort nested like a mosquito bite on a distant part of his back—itchy, but just out of reach, impossible to see.

Despite not being able to choose his university or his field of study, Samuel felt the freedom of university as a balm. He didn't relish engineering, but he was able to pursue his love of gospel music for the first time, listening to any album he chose, recording at local music studios, even cutting his first album. He earned enough money to cover his rent and tuition by writing election jingles for various political parties and sound tracks for home videos.

But the university—like all the others in southern Nigeria—was dominated by the cults. The cults had started as fraternities; it was Nigeria's sole Nobel Laureate, Wole Soyinka, who'd helped found the very first university group in 1952: the Pyrates Confraternity. These "pirates" sought to challenge the authorities for more freedoms. But over the years, pranks turned serious, petty crime grew rampant. Run-of-the-mill hooligans infiltrated the ranks, sensing opportunities for black-market activity. Carjackings and armed robberies abounded, and the minimal response by the police confirmed citizens' suspicions that the police were in cahoots with the criminals or, at the very least, so corrupt that they were bribed off with ease.

During the 1980s and '90s, the government used the fraternities as proxies to confront pro-democracy student groups during elections. Orchestrated protests escalated to ballot-box theft and eventually to assassination of opposition candidates.

The fraternities became known as cults, and they quickly staked out their territories. They intimidated students into joining with bullying, beatings, and arson. They harassed professors to provide good grades, storming into classrooms to strip professors of their clothing in front of their students. After several professors were summarily murdered in their classrooms, faculty members began swearing their own allegiance to cults.

But for all of their bravado and violence, the cults were leery of one group of students: the devout evangelical Christians. The cult members themselves had largely renounced religion—Catholicism, Protestantism, Islam, and native religions alike—but spiritual traditions were deeply ingrained in Nigerian society and held great sway. When Samuel was approached by the cults and responded by reading to them from his Bible, they backed off.

Samuel kept his opposition to the cults low-key. He wanted to befriend cult members, persuade them to renounce the cults and then convert to Christianity. Anyone who renounced cult membership immediately placed his life in danger, so this was a delicate process.

The Reverend Nwanko's style was different. He was vocal in his disdain for cults and avid in his desire to claim more lives for Christ. On visits home, Samuel dutifully acted as the pastor's son, but he wished that his father would assume a less bellicose posture. Such discussion or suggestion, however, was not an option.

In January, just before the arrival of the rains that marked the end of the brief dry season, Rev. Nwanko scored a coup—he helped the cousin of the governor of a neighboring state leave his cult and come to Jesus. This cousin not only renounced his cult but revealed names of its high-ranking members. A scandal quickly ignited, spreading through the news media, jeopardizing the governor's ability to run in the upcoming election.

Within a month, Rev. Nwanko's car was burned. A week later, cult members barged into his office and chased him out with sticks and bats. Then the reverend received a threat that "none of his children would have the chance to complete school." His daughters were married, not in university, so presumably they weren't the targets of this threat. The oldest son was studying abroad, so he was safe. The youngest was at a local university in Imo State; Rev. Nwanko told him to leave immediately and travel to relatives in another state.

Samuel, the middle son, was six hours away in Rivers State. Phone service in Nigeria had never been especially reliable, and Rev. Nwanko couldn't get through. Or at least, that's what he told Samuel much later.

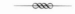

Samuel awoke in a hospital, floating in what seemed like a trance. Details of the assault drifted randomly back into his consciousness like tufts of cotton. For nine months he recovered in secrecy; the reason for his attack was withheld from him, and the fact of his survival withheld from the public. A guard was posted at the door, both to prevent suicide—Samuel made four attempts during his recuperation—and to prevent visitors. If it was known that Samuel had survived, his family reasoned, there could be violent retribution. And if Samuel knew that this had been an attack by the cults, not a random robbery...Well, his family couldn't be sure of the repercussions, so they felt it best not to correct his assumption.

The Nigerian doctors operated to repair Samuel's esophagus, which had been burned away by the sulfuric acid, but they did not possess the sophisticated plastic surgery techniques to address the extensive facial and retinal burns. For nine months Samuel lay in the hospital bed, swathed in gauze dressings, unmoored from the rest of society. The cruelest torture was eternal daylight. Without eyelids he was unable to sleep; the light bore down on him even through the dressings.

It was the cows that drew his attention to the news story that September. A cow was extremely valuable in Nigeria—the proceeds from selling a single cow could enable a person to purchase two cars. So when an Air France plane mowed down seven cows during a botched landing in Lagos, it was headline news. Samuel read every word of the story. The report listed some of the international notables who'd been on that plane—all, thankfully, uninjured. Buried in the fine print was the name of an American executive who worked for a charitable organization that brought patients with severe medical problems to America for treatment.

Samuel immediately e-mailed the agency and was dumbfounded to receive a reply just a few hours later: although the selection from Nigeria had already been made—a young girl from the countryside with severe cleft palate and facial deformities—they were willing to add a second case. Samuel called in his family and demanded to be discharged from the hospital that very day.

That was when Rev. Nwanko finally told his son the whole story: about the cousin of the governor who had renounced the cult, about being chased from his office by cult members, about the threats to his children, about trying—unsuccessfully, it seemed—to telephone Samuel to warn him.

The revelation of the truth behind the attack was less shocking to Samuel than the discussion itself. This was the first time in his life that Samuel had ever experienced his father talking to him like that—being honest, confessing fear, admitting error. The shock of this was overwhelming.

When the facts finally settled into him, Samuel expected to be overcome with fury toward his father, blaming him for the attack, castigating him for not trying harder to warn him about the threat. Was his life expendable, a mere trifle in the greater drive of his father's righteous zeal?

But the anger did not arise, at least not toward his father. Samuel was angry, yes, that this had derailed his graduation and wedding plans. But in his heart, he was convinced that this had been his destiny, that God knew from the moment he was born that this attack would happen. His father was not to blame.

Within a month Samuel was standing in the chaos of the Lagos airport preparing to fly to Buffalo, New York. His vision, which had been severely compromised by the attack, gave out altogether in the stress of the airport. The village girl with the cleft lip spoke no English. Her native language was barely intelligible because of her deformity, and she was terrified to be in the big city. So the two of them clung to each other in the vast, frenzied airport—she was the eyes, he the voice.

Once in Buffalo, Samuel underwent six surgeries to begin the long repair process. Skin patches were taken from his thighs and grafted onto his face and neck—an excruciating and arduous ordeal. There were many more surgeries that were needed, but he felt safe, for the first time in a year.

The agreement was that he could stay for four months for the surgeries, but then he had to return to his home country. This was the stipulation of his visa and also of the agency. Shortly before his scheduled return, however, Samuel met with an immigration lawyer to inquire about political asylum. The lawyer advised him that if he wanted to apply for political asylum he had to remain in the United States. Samuel wanted nothing more than to be rid of Nigeria, to be rid of Africa, to be rid of his past. The forms didn't seem difficult really, and the lawyer said he'd have a good chance.

But if he broke his initial agreement and chose to stay in America, the agency would not be permitted to select another patient from Nigeria. Samuel's freedom would cost the health of another of his fellow citizens. The guilt was too much for him. Besides, the cold weather in Buffalo was a constant irritant to the skin grafts on his face.

At the end of January, Samuel embarked on the most unbearable trip of his life, returning to the country of his attack. For the next year he remained holed up in his parents' house, fearing retaliation and violence. Only his family knew that he was there or even that he was alive. When guests were visiting, Samuel was confined to his bedroom, not even allowed to speak or laugh because the walls were so thin.

It was like he was back on that floor again, the flesh of his body pummeled into oblivion—only now it was his soul that was pummeled. The bleakness of his life was more painful than the attack. Samuel did nothing but sit in his room and stare at the flaking and water-stained plaster walls. When he could marshal some remnants of his spirit, he wrote letters to charitable organizations requesting help. On his better days, he trawled the Web for plastic surgeons anywhere in the world and e-mailed them to describe his case, hoping someone might offer the medical care he needed. Most days, though, he simply drew the blankets over his head. Darkness was preferable.

Alaba visited, but their contact was awkward. He knew that she couldn't wait for him to complete his medical treatments, that if she didn't marry within a year or two she'd be considered a spinster. Though he couldn't bear to look in the mirror, he knew that he didn't remotely resemble the man he'd been. He couldn't bring himself to ask whether she still wanted him. They ended their relationship by mutual agreement, but he knew she had just needed a graceful way out.

After a year of this subterranean existence, a surgeon on Long Island responded to one of his e-mails. If Samuel could cover his living expenses, this surgeon would perform the surgeries without charge. But living expenses in America were manyfold higher than in Nigeria, and there was the airline ticket too. This was more money than Rev. Nwanko's preaching brought in. It wouldn't be possible to do a fund-raising campaign, since Samuel's very existence was a secret. There was only one way Samuel could think of to raise money without revealing to anyone in Nigeria that he was alive—cutting an album.

Covering his face with a loose linen handkerchief, wearing a felt hat with a large, protruding brim, Samuel traveled to a recording studio in a far-flung town. He revealed his private agony for the first time in the only manner he could—singing to an anonymous microphone in a soundproof studio. He poured out all that he was able, crying in a way that only his music could offer, cloaking it all under a stage name. The three thousand dollars in CD sales was just enough to land him in the suburban bliss of Patchogue, Long Island.

⸺✖⸻

When Samuel Nwanko finished the story, my mouth felt parched. It was a burning dryness that snaked up into my head and burrowed into my stomach. A silence weighed between us. It slowly came to me that his story was completed, and that now it was my turn to take the reins of the conversation. I reached for the cup of water

I usually kept on my desk, but it was empty. "Wh-what," I finally stammered, "what are your main concerns right now?"

"Career training," Mr. Nwanko said, without missing a beat. "I must matriculate into university so I can finish my degree."

The ordinariness of his concerns took me aback. I guess I'd expected his main concerns to be about his injuries and their repair; how could he focus on anything else? But maybe it made perfect sense for him to focus on something else.

I trained my gaze on him as I performed a physical exam, trying to remain dispassionate, the neutral clinical observer, as I noted the nature and extent of the chemical burns on his face, neck, chest, back, and arms. H_2SO_4 is a potent acid that recklessly denatures proteins in its path. When combined with water, such as that contained in the cells of the human body, it produces a blast of heat. Sulfuric acid melts skin and muscle in a process called coagulation necrosis. This is as horrible as it sounds, but it has a saving grace: the dead tissue formed by the coagulation acts as a barrier to further acid penetration. Had Samuel's attackers used alkali rather than acid, the lipid strongholds of the tissue would have melted away as well—liquefaction necrosis—and the caustic agent would have seeped even deeper into the muscles and bones of his face.

I completed our visit with referrals to the ophthalmology clinic and the social worker, but I knew that Mr. Nwanko was not satisfied with this medical encounter. I wasn't either, but I didn't think that I or our system could offer him what he needed.

For the rest of the day, I was edgy. My temper was short, and I could not settle into a smooth groove of work. Whenever I reached for a glass of water, I winced. Even that night, I was restless, unable to find a comfortable position despite my fatigue. When I finally fell into an uneasy sleep, I dreamed of reaching a clear mountain stream after a strenuous hike. The water was clear, menacing. I was too afraid to drink.

———⋈———

Con intimo sentimento was how the largo movement was marked. Intimate sentiment—what exactly was that? The sentiment of the composer? The sentiment of the audience? The sentiment of the cellist?

I slid out the endpin of the cello and tightened the hairs on the bow. After a few strokes of rosin, I set about to coordinate the elements—left-hand fingers seeking the correct position on the fingerboard, right hand balancing the bow with simultaneous firmness and looseness, knees balancing the body of the instrument, ears straining to calibrate the intonation, eyes squinting at the scatter of notes on the page, brain juggling key signature, sharps, flats, rhythm, tone, bow direction, dynamics, then a quick consideration of *intimo sentimento*—and if I was lucky, I'd produce one single note.

Tuesdays I did not work in the hospital. Tuesday mornings I devoted to writing, and Tuesday afternoons were my cello lessons. The chaos of Mondays came to a screeching halt on Tuesdays.

I had started playing cello more out of parental duty than inclination, nipping onto an offhand piece of pedagogical advice when my daughter Naava started violin lessons. Predicting ferocious battles with my strong-willed child, I asked the teacher what was the best way to coax her into practicing. The teacher wiped the excess rosin off her violin strings with a soft cloth and replied, "The best thing for a child is to see a parent practicing."

I hailed the nearest taxi and promptly purchased a cheap Chinese-factory-made cello. I started lessons, applying the same brute-force approach I'd acquired in medical school—playing the same notes over and over again till they were seared in my memory like the Krebs cycle and the cranial nerves. But over time the cello ceased to be a parental device to influence my daughter's practice and grew to be my own musical journey.

This Tuesday I was working on Vivaldi's fifth cello sonata. I'd been plugging painfully through this piece, measure by measure, for almost a year now. We were up to the largo movement—*largo doloroso,* to be exact—and the editor had marked it *con intimo sentimento.*

I tried to think beyond the mechanics of playing to the intimate sentiment of the music, but all I could see was the disfigured face of Samuel Nwanko. The music was indeed slow and sad—*largo, doloroso*. The rich, melodic tones in B minor stretched painfully across measures, allowing ample time for reverberation and contemplation. When played by more competent hands than mine, the cello seemed to weep during this movement. When I thought of Mr. Nwanko, that was what I wanted to do. I wasn't able to fall in with his pragmatic optimism for the future—I just wanted to grieve over what had been stolen from him. I couldn't ever know the *intimo sentimento* of Antonio Vivaldi in the 1730s—the same years in which Bellevue Hospital first opened its doors—but three centuries later, his Baroque lament from Venice exactly captured my sadness about this young Nigerian man.

∽ Chapter Three ∽

Dr. Chan and Mrs. Geng eased out of their chairs in the waiting room using their matching wooden canes, the kind distributed by the hospital free of charge. At eighty-nine, Dr. Chan was stooped and frail, his body paper-thin. He seemed as though he might topple over from the breeze generated by the opening and closing of the clinic door. A translucent red plastic shopping bag from a Chinatown market dangled, as always, from one wrist. His other hand rested behind the elbow of his wife, not for his support, but so he could assist her. Mrs. Geng was younger by more than fifteen years and far more robust-appearing, but her progressing Alzheimer's disease and his stalwart chivalrousness made Dr. Chan the caregiver. He even carried her beige vinyl purse for her. Their clothes were worn, almost threadbare, but clean, pressed, and always layered for warmth.

Despite two decades in this country, Mrs. Geng spoke few words in English; her husband translated for her. Dr. Chan, who had been a cardiologist in China, spoke heavily accented, formal English in a whispery, halting voice. His utterances surfaced in brief puffs, with gaps in between that seemed to reflect the effort that English required. His voice felt as translucent as the shopping bag he always toted with him. I had to strain just to hear his words, and even more to extract the meaning from the tangle of his accent. But it was always worth the effort, because without fail I uncovered intelligently structured diction, with a dry wit to boot. Dr. Chan once told me that his English teacher in China taught only Shakespeare, and his German teacher only Goethe. "Not...very practical," he observed, in his studiously parsed syllables.

Dr. Chan and his wife shuffled into my office as I hurriedly tore off the wrinkled paper on the exam table left from the previous patient. It was one of those sessions in which everything and everyone was running late. But there was no cutting corners with Dr. Chan—he moved at his methodical pace, spoke in his measured phrasing. Plus, it was always two patient visits in one, as I had both husband and wife to treat.

Dr. Chan carefully laid a sheet of lined paper, torn from a spiral notebook, onto my desk. On the paper were four columns of hand-printed figures—blood-pressure and glucose values for both Dr. Chan and Mrs. Geng for the past three months. This was how every visit with them started.

Dr. Chan and Mrs. Geng had emigrated from China later in life than most immigrants. Dr. Chan was then seventy-one and had just retired from medicine. His brother, who'd already been living in the United States, encouraged them to come, boasting of the wonderful American life. He helped them to obtain their temporary visas and even contributed to the plane fares.

At first, Dr. Chan opened a storefront clinic on East Broadway, selling herbs and offering Chinese medicine to local residents. Many immigrants were fearful of American hospitals and would go only to herbalists. For years Dr. Chan quietly triaged patients from behind his display counter of herbs, spotting goiters and cardiomyopathies, convincing the patrons that a visit to a Western doctor would not conflict with Eastern medicine.

He stayed in the clinic until he was almost eighty. During those years, he and Mrs. Geng worked patiently through the immigration system to obtain their green cards. His older brother had died in the interim, so Dr. Chan did the paperwork himself. Once he was a legal immigrant he was able to earn a small salary from his clinic. They began the daunting process of applying for citizenship. Older and significantly frailer by then, Dr. Chan finally closed the clinic and moved with his wife into housing for the elderly, a building that happened to be located precisely across the street from where I lived.

The first time I glanced at Dr. Chan's chart I did a double take— I thought I was seeing my own address printed there. Our building numbers were only one digit apart, and our apartments were both on the fifth floor. Our addresses were nearly indistinguishable, but I didn't think it proper to point this out.

Eventually, however, I started running into them on the street while I was out with my children or walking our dog. Rather than being embarrassed by our proximity, Dr. Chan commented, "Not only...do we have...good doctor...we also have...good neighbor."

Mrs. Geng had grown more forgetful over the years, and this was distressing to her husband. He took care of her assiduously, and she was always well groomed, with perfect skin and hygiene.

Despite his good care, however, Mrs. Geng had been losing weight. Dr. Chan cooked three meals a day for her and made sure that she ate. At each clinic visit, however, she was a kilogram less. "I cannot identify...the etiology," Dr. Chan told me. "I have observed...no rectal bleeding...no vaginal discharge. She has no...thyromegaly. I cannot palpate...her spleen...nor her liver. She has no irregular...heart rhythms. Her glucose level...remains normal."

Routine blood tests revealed nothing grossly amiss. We talked about a more extensive workup, but Mrs. Geng declined. Dr. Chan nodded in agreement. We both understood the grim course of Alzheimer's that lay ahead for Mrs. Geng. The treatment of any disease or cancer that might be found would involve much physical hardship and likely limited gain for a woman who was destined to lose her awareness and control of most bodily functions in the coming years.

Today, Dr. Chan had a different concern. "I must report," he said, resting his cane on the back of the chair, "a decrease in frequency...of bowel function. Evacuation is...extremely difficult."

"Have you always been constipated," I asked, "or is this something recent?"

"Oh, many years," he said. "Ever since...I move to America."

I wondered if this was due to a change in diet, but Dr. Chan insisted that he consumed exactly the same diet as in China. Weekly trips to the markets in Chinatown ensured that he could obtain the same vegetables, herbs, spices, and oils that he'd grown up with.

"Life in China...regular," Dr. Chan said. "Life in America... irregular."

I commiserated with him, commenting that there wasn't much we could do to change the rhythms of life in America but that there were treatments for constipation that we could offer.

"I take...laxative, everything," he said, shaking his head. "But still...I cannot...expel it. Sometimes my wife...has to disimpact...for me." Dr. Chan said this without pause, without shame. He simply stated the fact, now that I'd asked. His wife, who couldn't follow our English, was unaware of what he was saying.

I, on the other hand, was struck by this. Was this humiliating for Dr. Chan? Was it uncomfortable to ask her? "No," he replied matter-of-factly. "She was...nurse."

In the three years that I'd known him I hadn't been aware of the degree to which this "minor" medical issue dictated his day-to-day life. I hadn't asked about it, and he hadn't volunteered it.

I had also underestimated Mrs. Geng's abilities. I'd thought of her as the typical passive Alzheimer's patient, like a docile child, being cared for by her husband and the part-time home attendant. I could see now that the language barriers had reinforced a misconception.

But what I found most remarkable about this fragile immigrant couple was the intimacy of their care of each other in growing old. Dr. Chan and Mrs. Geng had married twenty-five years ago. Both had children from previous marriages; Dr. Chan's first wife had died of leukemia. But they had come together in the second half of adulthood, supporting each other through old age: frail Dr. Chan guiding his wife out of her chair; demented Mrs. Geng relieving her husband of his most painful symptoms. I watched them together in my exam room, Dr. Chan whispering translations of my instructions to his wife, Mrs. Geng gently touching her husband to ask a question. The two of them with their identical canes, the wooden veneers worn away at the handles where they gripped daily. They had truly intertwined their lives—neither could live, it seemed, without the other.

I feared for both. Dr. Chan—older and with more medical problems, easily liable to succumb before his wife. Mrs. Geng—carrying the albatross of Alzheimer's disease that could soon transform her into an incoherent, incontinent, uncommunicative woman.

Just four months earlier, we'd had a medical scare. Dr. Chan awoke one morning completely paralyzed on the left side of his body. He diagnosed his own ischemic stroke of the right middle cerebral artery and patiently explained the pathophysiology to the baffled 911 operator. He was rushed to Bellevue, admitted to the intensive care unit, but turned out to be one of the lucky ones whose symptoms resolved within twenty-four hours. In those twenty-four hours he managed to charm the paramedics, ER staff, neurology team, and orderlies with his unfailing politeness and his sweet, understated personality, which came through despite his labored, accented English. His stroke was downgraded to a TIA (transient ischemic attack) and he was discharged a few days later with two antiplatelet agents added to his drug regimen but otherwise no worse for the wear. But had he remained paralyzed, he and his wife both would likely be in nursing homes now.

I believed that this was what Dr. Chan feared—that he'd get sick first, that he'd be unable to care for his wife, that they'd end up in separate nursing homes. The tenuous balance of their lives scared me—their medical, financial, social, and linguistic precariousness. I'd spoken with them extensively about advance directives. Both stated that they'd never want to be on life-support machines. I documented this in their medical records as clearly as I could, knowing that their communication powers were limited.

I was sure that their truest wish was that they'd die together, that neither would leave the other alone, unattended. But I couldn't put that in the advance-directive form. I could only hope that this would be the way it would turn out. Then I did something I rarely did with my other patients—I gave Dr. Chan my personal cell phone number. "If anything serious ever happens," I said, "please call me."

I stared at my notes about their advance-directive wishes, realizing that I might be the only person in possession of this information. If the worst happened, I'd be the one to testify that they did not want invasive procedures. I might be the one signing their DNRs.

When our appointment finished, I held the door for Dr. Chan and Mrs. Geng, then watched them walk down the hall to the elevators. Frail Dr. Chan shuffled, leaning heavily on his cane. He hunched over as he walked, appearing to stare at the ground. But he clasped his wife's elbow the whole way. Mrs. Geng used her cane more as a marker for her steps than anything else. She stood upright, solid in her movements. To the outsider's eye, it seemed that Mrs. Geng was supporting Dr. Chan. But I knew that he was attempting to do the reverse, even if it wasn't altogether possible.

After they'd left, I saw that Mrs. Uddin was already waiting for me, and I knew I'd never get through the morning session. Whoever invented the fifteen-minute patient slot had never met Nazma Uddin. Mrs. Uddin—a heavyset woman from Bangladesh—always had a thousand complaints, endless aches and pains, never-ending misery. Today she was wearing her usual dark blue heavy polyester robe, head scarf, and veil. Only her eyes and forehead were visible. But when I closed the door she immediately unsnapped the veil, and we smiled sympathetically at each other, gearing ourselves up for the inevitable frustrations that lay ahead. At this point in our relationship, however, a visit with her did not unnerve me. But it hadn't always been that way. She used to be my torment.

I had first become Mrs. Uddin's doctor eight years before. She was only thirty-five years old, but she'd seemed so aged and infirm that it shocked me to see that we were the same age. Each visit was an endless litany of hiccups, headaches, shin pains, stomach pains, ear pains, coccyx pains. Despite innumerable CT scans, blood tests, specialty consultations, cardiac stress tests, lung function tests, endoscopies, and MRIs, there was nothing concrete I could find to explain her complaints. No therapy I offered seemed to help. There was clearly a psychological element to her condition, but she never followed through with referrals to psychiatrists or trials of antidepressant medications. She had some amorphous blend of chronic pain syndrome, osteoarthritis, fibromyalgia, depression, dyspepsia, somatization disorder, migraines, stress—all of which I treated. But nothing ever got better. I dreaded her visits.

In those years, Mrs. Uddin always brought along her young daughter, Azina—a solemn, bespectacled girl with a round face that was accentuated by the flowered head scarf pinned under her chin. Mrs. Uddin droned on in Bengali about the needlelike pains in her ears, the fire feeling in her head, the bursting veins in her intestines, the bad air that was stuck inside her lungs. Azina sat hunched on my exam table, glumly translating while I scanned the computer, disheartened at the inordinate amount of medical testing Mrs. Uddin had undergone.

I was annoyed that Mrs. Uddin kept Azina out of school for these appointments. I was exasperated by her extravagant overuse of the medical system. I always felt as though I were going to drown in Mrs. Uddin's unremitting complaints, as though she were deliberately trying to torture me with her unsolvable issues. If I didn't control my feelings, my mind would spin with frustration, perseverating about how much I hated the whine in her voice, hated seeing her name on my roster, hated the fact that she'd emigrated thousands of miles from some random village in Bangladesh and had somehow managed to end up in *my* clinic with her intractable and dispiriting medical complaints. And especially about how much I hated that stultifying, dehumanizing veil.

The tension between us finally broke one day when Azina piped up and asked if we were done yet because she wanted to get back to school in time for recess. The shock of her own voice and her own words was like ice water. I realized that I had slipped too far in my own irrational feelings, that my anger was flagrantly displaced, and that I had lost all sense of the humanity of my patient and her daughter.

Azina quietly told me what it was like at home with a mother who was depressed and in pain, how the burden of caring for her mother and the family had fallen on her shoulders, how she ached to just worry about homework, like the rest of the fifth-graders. This revelation opened my eyes and helped me regain my empathy—and energy—for Mrs. Uddin. After that, I no longer saw Mrs. Uddin as a torment; Azina had cured me of that.

Today Mrs. Uddin was here with her usual complaints, none of which had changed—or progressed—since we'd first met. Over the years, we'd acquired a familiarity with each other's quirks, and in some ways we felt like an old married couple. Her English had improved, and she was able to negotiate her health care largely on her own. I had made her promise not to take Azina out of school anymore, and she'd remained faithful to that agreement.

I nodded as Mrs. Uddin spoke about her scalp splitting in two, her appetite that tolerated only boiled okra, her knees that cracked open on the stairs, her spine that curved to the left. I noted all her aches and pains in the chart, but somehow they didn't feel like assaults on my being as they used to. It was easier now—now that we knew each other so well—to sort through the morass, to keep it from suffocating me. Our visits still ran generously over the allotted fifteen minutes, but I no longer felt angry, thanks to the perspective that Azina had helped me with so many years ago.

I still had my own personal discomfort with the concept of the veil. The theme of finding women's bodies and sexuality threatening, something that needed to be controlled, seemed to be a commonality in so many cultures. My children were still young, but at some point they'd notice that in Orthodox Judaism, women had to sit behind a barrier in synagogue and were not participants in any of the ceremony. Later they might learn how menstruation supposedly rendered women "unclean." How was I going to explain these concepts to them?

However, I recognized that many Muslim women chose the veil voluntarily, as a symbol of piety, modesty, and perhaps as a way to shield their personal lives from the outside world. So, too, many Orthodox Jewish women chose their role voluntarily and felt no qualms about segregated seating or covering their hair. I had to respect that, though I was sure there were some women in both religions who felt coerced. Still, I needed to keep my political and feminist concerns out of my individual encounters with women who wore the veil. Nazma Uddin wore it, and my years of treating her had gone a long way toward making me more comfortable with the veil.

I didn't have any solutions for Mrs. Uddin today, but the very act of unloading her concerns seemed to relax her. I offered my sympathy for her pains. I suggested that we try physical therapy again. I reminded her that weight loss would help her aching knees.

I recommended that she consider acupuncture—she'd always been leery about that one—and I refilled her panoply of prescriptions. I convinced her to give the antidepressants another try. She assented this time, but I knew there was only a fifty-fifty chance that she'd take them.

She snapped her veil back on and stood to go. We gave each other a hug, as we always did now. We had a lot of years behind us, and it was clear that we had a lot ahead of us too.

◇ Chapter Four ◇

"'Julia Barquero is a thirty-six-year-old Guatemalan female with an exacerbation of congestive heart failure,'" the intern recited from her index card. We were on rounds, getting to know all of our new patients on the first day of the month. Most of my time was spent in the outpatient clinic of Bellevue, but for three months each year I worked full-time on the inpatient medical wards supervising a team of residents, interns, and medical students.

Inpatient medicine had a different rhythm than outpatient medicine. On the surface, it was more active—sicker patients, acute illnesses, rounding on patients spread throughout the hospital, going up and down the elevators to the ER, to radiology, to the prison ward. But strangely enough, it felt less discombobulating than the clinic. Clinic, with its ostensibly less ill patients, was traditionally considered to be the milder of milieus; in fact, it was an open-ended maelstrom of ceaseless patients, desultory and scattershot clinical conundrums, never-ending time crunches, plus chaotic scheduling that led to a different medley of interns and residents each day whose names I could never hope to master.

In contrast, on the inpatient wards, we were a single tightly knit team, working together every day, all day, for four straight weeks. We took care of the patients together, tackled the problems together, learned together. I ran teaching rounds with the same group of residents and interns every day. It felt like the ideal of academic medicine.

But the most significant difference compared to the outpatient clinic was that our clinical responsibilities were clearly circumscribed. No matter how hairy things got, nothing ever extended beyond the specific patients assigned to our service. These patients—and *only* these patients—were our responsibility, and this ability to focus was a luxury I could only dream about when I was in clinic.

Now I looked quizzically at the team. Usually, congestive heart failure was the purview of seventy-six-year-olds, not thirty-six-year-olds. The resident on the team was a Filipino who'd been raised in Cleveland, and his flat midwestern accent never ceased to elicit a chuckle from those who didn't know him. But I always enjoyed rounds with him because of his impressive fund of knowledge coupled with an utter absence of obnoxious ego. He pulled the echocardiogram report from where it had been stashed in his copy of the most recent *Annals of Internal Medicine,* and he walked his interns and students through it.

According to the echocardiogram, Julia Barquero's heart was barely pumping. It hadn't been battered by multiple heart attacks, as the typical seventy-six-year-old heart patient's was; instead, she had a dilated cardiomyopathy—all chambers of the heart were smoothly and equally distended. Maybe she'd contracted an infection of her heart as a child in Guatemala, or maybe she'd inherited a genetic glitch—at this point, the cause was irrelevant. The overstretched muscle fibers could not muster enough force for the usual crisp squeeze of the heart that sent a quarter cup of blood shooting through the body's arterial tree eighty times per minute. Instead, each beat of Julia Barquero's heart was a flaccid hiccup that dribbled out just a tablespoon of oxygenated blood. The body could compensate for this limited outflow by increasing the heart rate and tightening the vessels, but eventually these physiologic compromises failed and fluid backed up into the legs and lungs—the symptoms of congestive heart failure.

According to the chart, the intern reported, the patient had been diagnosed only recently with dilated cardiomyopathy, when increasing shortness of breath had forced her into a local hospital in Brooklyn. After a four-month stay, she'd been discharged with a clutch of medicines to help stabilize her fluid balance. These helped, but she had come to Bellevue because she was still feeling under the weather and her friends had told her that Bellevue was a better hospital for heart problems.

The intern pushed loose hair away from her forehead as she spoke. She was a tall, sinewy woman of Indian descent with implacably curious obsidian eyes and a reticent mien who towered over her squatly built resident. Although our team had been together for only three hours, the resident had already started loosening her up with his steady commentary about the brevity of his NBA career and the first prize he'd taken in the annual Filipino gnome contest.

The intern cleared her throat and turned over her index card. "The report from the previous team is that she's pretty much tuned up," she said as we entered the room. "Just about ready to go."

The two hospital beds in the room were both occupied by young, Hispanic-looking women. "Julia Barquero?" I asked, looking from bed to bed.

"*Hoo-li-yah,*" the woman in the bed by the window politely corrected me.

I winced because I should have known better—in Spanish, a *j* is pronounced like an *h*. My Spanish education over the years had been piecemeal—a summer class in Oaxaca, a two-week language school in Peru, a week during a vacation in Guatemala—and although I could speak a modest amount of Spanish to my patients, I still constantly made errors.

"*Julia,*" I said again, this time pronouncing it correctly, and I was rewarded with an unprepossessing smile.

Julia Barquero was a slight woman sitting up on the edge of the bed with a back issue of *Vanidades* from the mobile patient library in her lap. Thick black bangs reached low on her forehead, dusting the edges of her eyebrows, camouflaging a scattering of leftover acne. She had a youthful appearance, but I could see the exhaustion from her hospitalization in the tea-colored bags under her eyes.

Julia was breathing comfortably and had no edema in her legs. When we listened to her lungs, there wasn't a speck of congestion. With the help of medications, her otherwise healthy body was compensating effectively and invisibly for her failing heart; to look at her you would never know.

But I knew. We all knew. Dilated cardiomyopathies did not get better. Her only chance was a heart transplant.

"She's undocumented," the intern said sotto voce, and not another word needed to pass between us. Julia's fate was sealed. Undocumented patients—illegal aliens—couldn't get on the transplant list.

Down the hall we came to our next patient. The intern pulled out another index card and read mechanically, "'Amadou Sow is a forty-nine-year-old man from Senegal. He was admitted a week ago with lung cancer, metastatic to his bones. Oncology feels that the best treatment for him is radiation to palliate his pain.'"

The resident interrupted. "It's a disposition issue," he said. "Radiation therapy is outpatient treatment—daily for thirty days. The hospital wants him discharged, because if he stays they won't get reimbursed for what should be outpatient treatment. Problem is, he needs an ambulette to bring him to and from the outpatient radiation. But he's undocumented, so he doesn't qualify for any services."

"Could he get to the treatment by bus?" I asked.

"Well, that's the problem," said the resident, balling his hands into fists in his pockets. "He can't walk because of the mets in his bones. Plus he lives in a fourth-floor walk-up."

We entered the room. Amadou Sow was lying in bed, but the head of the bed was raised to the highest level, so he was nearly sitting up. He was long and willowy, his limbs unfurling like vines.

"Greetings, Doctors," he said cheerfully. His voice was robust, lilted with a heavy West African accent. His eyes were quick, taking each of us in, one at a time.

"Good morning, Mr. Sow," I said. "I'm Dr. Ofri and this is the new medical team who will be taking care of you." He sat forward and patiently allowed us to listen to his heart and lungs, multiple stethoscopes crisscrossing his body.

"Are you having any pain now?" I asked.

"At the moment, not too much," Mr. Sow replied. "The morphine is at the right level. But they say that the radiation will help the pain get better, so I am looking forward to starting next week."

The resident raised his eyebrows to me, then edged discreetly out of the way.

"What do you understand about the radiation treatments, Mr. Sow?" I asked.

His eyes caught mine and his voice grew sober. "I know that the hospital wants to send me home to do the treatments. The person has already come to tell me that." Then he cocked his head to one side. "But I understand," he said forthrightly. "You shouldn't have to pay for me. I want to go to my home. I don't want to see these bills go any higher."

"You are right that it is expensive to stay in the hospital," I said, "but there are other options, like a nursing home or a hospice—"

"No, no." He cut me off with a pained wave of his gangly arm. "I need to go to my apartment. Whatever time I have left I must have with my wife and children."

"But is that realistic?" I asked. "How will you get up and down four flights of steps?"

"My children will help me," he said with a broad smile. "They are strong boys."

"How old are they?" I asked.

"Eight and ten."

The next day was Julia's discharge. The intern and I stood at her bedside reviewing the list of medications with her. Julia sat on the edge of her neatly made bed. I pointed to each medication on the list and explained in simple Spanish that the diuretic worked to get rid of water, the beta-blocker made the heart need less oxygen, the ACE inhibitor relaxed the blood vessels, and the digoxin made the heart muscle work better.

"¿Cuánto cuestan estas medicinas?" Julia asked. Her voice had a faint huskiness to it, as though she breathed around her words to keep them afloat.

"There isn't any extra charge for the medicines you get when you leave the hospital," I said, "but when you refill the medicines at the pharmacy there is a co-pay of ten dollars for each prescription."

Julia's brow furrowed and her lips moved silently as she appeared to be doing a mental calculation. "Every month?" she asked. I nodded. There was a pause as she cogitated some more. Then her face went slack. Her right hand reached down to the sheet on her bed, straightening it even though it was already perfectly tucked in.

"Do I need *all* of the pills?" she asked. The intern raised her eyes to me.

"Yes," I said. "Unfortunately you do."

"Will they make me better?"

"They will make you feel better," I replied. "They will keep out the extra water and help your heart work."

"But will they make me *better*?" she repeated, her hand leaving the sheet and reaching up to curl her hair with an index finger.

"Better?" I stopped to consider my words. I had a limited repertoire in Spanish. I could say the basics, but I couldn't—as I would normally do in English in such a situation—rephrase what I was saying or use a metaphor or describe shades of gray. I certainly couldn't massage my words to beat around the bush. "The medicines will stabilize your heart. They will make you feel better."

"But will I get *better*?" Julia's voice was straightforward, not accusing or second-guessing. The intern shuffled and looked down to the floor.

Of course Julia knew. She'd spent four months at the hospital in Brooklyn. She had to know. So I explained again about the medicines, rotating my finite stock of Spanish phrases, hedging about how the medications would control the symptoms and keep everything in balance.

When she asked a fourth time, I began to think that perhaps Julia really did not understand the full nature of her illness. Could it be that the doctors who'd made the diagnosis had not fully explained the prognosis? Or had Julia been unable, or unwilling, to absorb the facts?

The intern at my side was nervously twisting her stethoscope, keeping her gaze locked on the tips of her sneakers. The patient in the next bed over was listening, following our conversation with the bizarre intimacy that hospital rooms produced. I wanted to do the right thing, as a doctor, teacher, role model.

But even if I'd possessed the sophistication in Spanish, how could I possibly have said to a thirty-six-year-old that there existed a cure for her condition but that for reasons entirely unmedical it was unavailable to her, and that soon even the solid youthfulness of her body would no longer compensate. That the muscles of her heart would falter, fluid would choke her lungs, and she would become an old woman quickly—hobbling, gasping, spending more time in the hospital than in her home. That the end would be brutal and protracted, and that she would likely not live to see forty-six. That had random chance caused her to be born on this side of the border, she might have had a shot at seeing her children enter middle school.

I stammered another iteration about the medicines helping the heart and slunk out of the room. I'd failed Julia as a doctor, and I'd failed my intern as a teacher. I'd chickened out, and I knew it.

After lunch, I went back to Julia's room alone, determined to be straight with her. She was standing by the window, fully dressed. From the sixteenth-floor window, all of downtown Manhattan was spread before us. The Williamsburg, Manhattan, and Brooklyn bridges stretched like lazy felines across the shimmering East River. But when I got closer, I saw that Julia wasn't looking at any of this spectacular scenery. Instead, she was staring at a dog-eared strip of black-and-white photos, the type from a photo booth. There were four shots of a somber-looking child with thick curly hair being held up by adult hands. He was turned this way and that for the photos, as if the adult were trying to get all angles of the boy.

"*Mi hijo,*" Julia said. "*Vasco.*"

"*¿Su hijo?*" I said. "*¿Aquí en Nueva York?*"

It was the way she shook her head, like a sagging pendulum that lingered painfully at each end of its arc, that strangled my prepared speech about her cardiomyopathy. We stood side by side at the window—she looking down at the photos, I looking out past the river. Her voice deepened to a contralto as she related her story.

When Vasco was only a few weeks old, he'd contracted meningitis and had been hospitalized for two months. He never was right after that, and the Guatemalan doctors couldn't help. Julia decided that she had to get him to America, that this was the only way to get him the medical care that he needed. Her husband had already traveled north to New York and was sending money when he could. Julia knew that it would be difficult to get across the border with a baby; she decided to go by herself and then try to bring him later, once she was established.

She left baby Vasco with her mother in the rural village in which she herself had been born. Julia walked for nearly eight weeks with coyotes—smugglers—through the length of Mexico, north to Texas. It took months, but she finally made her way to Brooklyn to meet her husband.

Once Julia arrived in New York she quickly found a night-shift job cleaning offices at Con Edison—apparently no one cared about working papers at that time of night. It turned out to be much harder to send for Vasco than she'd expected. Julia was heartbroken about not being able to see her son; if she traveled to Guatemala, it would be unlikely that she'd ever be able to return to the United States. In the meantime, she and her husband had a baby girl in New York. Her husband soon lost his construction job, so he followed the building boom to Florida to earn money there. Julia had continued working at Con Ed while raising Lucita until symptoms of breathlessness forced her to quit and seek medical attention.

Julia's son, Vasco, wasn't the only one in her family to face illness; in fact, it seemed that Julia's family had more than its fair share. First there was cancer. One of Julia's brothers died at age eighteen of a brain tumor. Another brother was living with lung cancer even though he had never smoked. One of her sisters died of ovarian cancer at age twenty-nine. Another sister developed ovarian cancer at age twenty-two, but it was discovered at an early stage and she was cured with surgery.

Then there were the heart problems. One of Julia's sisters died at age eighteen of a heart condition. Another brother also had a heart condition. And now, it seemed, Julia was next in line.

As I stood with Julia at the window, I suspected that she did have some awareness of her condition, but it was still my job to clarify the facts for her. I took a step back and gazed at her narrow figure outlined by the million-dollar Manhattan view. The concentric rings of sadness—for her son, for her siblings, for what seemed to be her genetic fate—were too potent to breach. I couldn't bear to add another layer. Once again, I edged shamefacedly out of the room. Julia left the hospital with only a brown paper bag full of pill bottles.

—⊶∞⊷—

Amadou Sow was ready for discharge at the end of the week. We convinced the hospital to at least provide a charity ambulette to return the patient to his home. The ambulette workers would not, of course, carry him up the stairs, but at least he would make it to his front door.

Our team was turning the corner at the far end of the ward when we saw Mr. Sow being bundled into a stretcher by the ambulette attendants. We stopped in front of him as the attendants tightened the neon orange seat belts around his silver-blanketed torso.

"I am ready for the space shuttle," Mr. Sow said with a lopsided grin.

We all chuckled, but our laughter petered out in a thin trail. We knew we were sending Mr. Sow into a shaky unknown. The odds were overwhelming that he'd never obtain the medical care he needed. In order for Mr. Sow to get to his daily radiation treatments, someone would have to carry him up and down four flights of stairs every single day. I imagined his wife supporting his right side with their sons on his left—the eight-year-old grasping the arm and the ten-year-old cradling the leg. They'd start at their apartment door, at the top of the narrow tenement stairs. They wouldn't be able to fit en masse in the stairwell, so they'd have to angle themselves, the wife going first, the children second, with Mr. Sow jiggling between them. His right side would jolt down a step with his wife, then his left would follow. Step by step, ratcheting down forty splintering wooden stairs.

Metastatic lesions in the bones offer deep-seated, boring pain, and patients learn early on that being still is safest. Mr. Sow, however, would keep silent during the jerking trip down the stairs, not wanting to inflict his own pain on his family. His sons would likewise remain silent, not wanting to let on how arduous the task was; even a cancer-worn body is heavy for little boys. Only his wife would speak during their daily journeys, with a steady stream of encouragements. When they rested at the tiny landings, she would recount stories from Senegal, as much to coax energy from her husband as to edify her children, who recalled little from their native land.

Once at the bottom of the stairs they'd ease their way out of the narrow landing. Luckily, the bus stop was only a block from their building, and with two transfers they could get to the hospital in ninety minutes. The radiation treatment itself only lasts a half hour, and then they'd do the whole thing in reverse. For one day, and then the next. Maybe the third. But how long could they continue? The four flights up were harder than the four flights down. The Sows couldn't keep their sons out of school indefinitely.

Eventually, it would defeat them. Just as the cancer was defeating Mr. Sow, so too would it defeat his family. Although they perhaps didn't comprehend the term *palliative,* they would at some point understand that the radiation wasn't going to cure his cancer, that he was going to die with or without it.

Hopefully his oncologist would have already given him morphine—adequate dose, adequate supply. Hopefully his family had plenty of pillows to protect the sore spots. Hopefully the sounds and smells of dying would not frighten his children. Hopefully his wife had a job that would allow her to support her family after his death. Hopefully their apartment wasn't located too close to the elevated train, so that his last hours would not be disturbed by the clattering subway.

All this we hoped for as his stretcher was rolled away. Mr. Sow gingerly lifted an arm to wave to us as the attendants wheeled him toward the elevator. We stood silently while the doors opened, took him in, and then closed again.

———⚉———

Julia Barquero had left the hospital without full knowledge of her medical condition. I was complicit in this act, along with the cardiology fellow and Julia's regular clinic doctor. I remembered watching the cardiologist—an intelligent, compassionate physician from Bulgaria—speak with Julia via an interpreter. Julia again asked if the medicines would make her better. The cardiologist didn't lie— she emphasized over and over again that the medicines were only to treat her symptoms—but she couldn't bring herself to speak the harsh words so directly any more than I could.

Why were we so scared to tell the truth? Looking back now, I know that there were many issues involved, but the overriding emotion was fear. We were each terrified of being the one to deliver the death sentence. If we'd been in a private hospital with an American citizen, we'd have been discussing the ways this disease could be cured. Of course we couldn't guarantee that the patient would definitely get a heart—plenty of people died on the waiting list—but at least there would have been some sort of beacon to yearn toward.

To a policymaker, it made perfect sense to limit organ donation to citizens only. On an intellectual level, we could appreciate this concept, even agree with it, but on a human level, it sapped our courage, leaving Julia far too long in the dark and her doctors with ongoing pangs of guilt.

Julia finally got the news a few weeks after she was discharged. She sat in the medical clinic with the resident, a freckled, dark-haired woman of Irish descent. The resident told me that she had explained to Julia, via an interpreter, that her heart was swollen and stretched. Julia had asked once again if the medicines would make her better. The resident paused, took a deep breath, and finally said it. "The medicines could help you feel better, but only a heart transplant could cure the condition." After an even longer pause she lowered her voice. "But we can't put you on the list because you are undocumented."

Julia hadn't flinched, or cried, or even blinked. She'd just stared straight ahead. After a few minutes, she gathered her pill bottles that had been lined up on the desk and tucked them in her purse. The resident handed her the new prescriptions, and the visit ended as any other visit might.

∽ Chapter Five ∽

Some weeks later, when I spotted the name Amadou Sow on my appointment roster in clinic, I was ecstatic: Mr. Sow had survived the trip home, and was well enough to return for a clinic visit. There was something about his infectious optimism that had kept me cherishing the secret hope that he'd prevail despite every depressing fact insisting otherwise. A true vindication of the human spirit.

So when a strapping hulk of a man strode into my office, I was crushed and had to struggle to conceal my disappointment. There were all sorts of John Does at Bellevue, and Amadou Sow was the John Doe of West Africa. I'd lost track of how many patients of mine were named Amadou Sow, Mamadou Sow, or Sow Amadou. This particular Amadou Sow was from Mali and spoke only Bambara and French. Reluctantly, I put aside my thoughts about the Amadou Sow from Senegal—who might already be dead, for all I knew—and focused on this new Amadou Sow, the robust young man from Mali.

A decade ago, a new patient who spoke only French would have been like a weight crushing my shoulders; I'd know that I'd have to spend more than half my allotted time with him scrambling for an interpreter. Fortunately, in the last few years, Bellevue had leaped into the modern age of language interpretation and hired simultaneous interpreters in the most common languages. They were secreted somewhere—maybe they weren't even in the hospital at all, who knew?—but all I had to do was pick up my phone and dial extension 1800.

"Welcome to the Medical Interpretation Service," the recorded voice would say. "Press one for Spanish. Press two for Mandarin. Press three for Cantonese. Press four for Fukianese. Press five for Bengali. Press pound one for Polish. Press pound two for French. Press pound three for Creole."

It's not that French was entirely foreign to me. I did study it in junior high school and even competed in the eighth-grade French spelling bee. Every time I had a West African patient I was tempted to try to speak French, but I was always reminded of my experience with Aristide Mezondes during one of my first years as an attending at Bellevue.

"*Je m-m'a . . . ,*" I'd stuttered to Mr. Mezondes, the serious young man in a gray wool overcoat standing before me with ramrod posture. "*Je m'appelle Dr. Ofri.*"

There. I'd gotten it out.

The language of Descartes, Voltaire, and Balzac had clearly vacated my cortex. Despite those years of French classes and one brief visit to Paris, *Je m'appelle* was the best I could come up with. And even that was a struggle. Pushed aside by the overwhelming necessity for Spanish in our clinic, further dilapidated by decades of disuse, my French shriveled until I could not conjure up a single word beyond stating my name. I was appalled at my brain's porosity.

Mr. Mezondes smiled politely. No doubt he was accustomed, and perhaps resigned, to the challenges of communication here in America. I gestured for him to sit and tried to signal a polite *just a moment* as I started down the list of options. First was calling the office of our volunteer interpreters.

"Sorry," the person who answered said, "our French interpreter is no longer with us." I hoped he had merely quit his job and not met an untimely end.

I asked around in the waiting room, but nobody spoke French. I canvassed the clinic staff—only Spanish and Chinese to be found. Back at my office, I resorted to the final option and called AT&T. When a French-accented voice graced my ear, I exhaled a sigh of relief.

Mr. Mezondes and I took turns on the phone, and I learned that he was twenty-four years old and from Braazaville in Congo. He spent an extra cycle of translation ensuring that I understood that this was the Congo that used to be French Congo, not the Congo that used to be Zaire. He was generally healthy, but his main concern was a burning in his stomach, especially after he ate.

Even though we smiled gamely at each other as we handed the phone back and forth, it was hard to say that we were really having a conversation. It was more like we were each having a conversation with the polite but businesslike interpreter. And that's what our conversation was: polite and businesslike. I asked the questions, he supplied the answers. I kept my utterances brief, not wishing to overload the operator, and I sensed Mr. Mezondes doing the same. I was also cognizant of the cost of the services, so I tried to be as efficient as possible. I even ventured to tell my patient his probable diagnosis and treatment during this initial conversation, something I normally would never do before the physical exam. But I didn't want to have to call the operator back, so I explained that he most likely had acid reflux, and—barring any information to the contrary that I might glean from the physical exam—that I would give him a medicine for acid and see him again in my clinic in one month.

We said good-bye to our AT&T friend and I gestured him up onto the exam table. As I palpated his abdomen and listened to his heart, Mr. Mezondes asked in halting English, "You speak little *français?*"

"No." I shook my head, regretting the years of study that had never succeeded in cementing my French. *"Solamente español."*

"¿Español?" he said with a broad grin. *"Yo hablo español."*

Spanish? He spoke Spanish?

For the rest of our visit, we chatted happily, if a bit awkwardly, in our mutual nonnative language. I learned that he'd studied Spanish at his university in Congo, and I told him that I'd studied on trips to Latin America.

He told me how he had emigrated from Africa two years ago but had first lived in Canada, and how different Canada was from America. I told him that I had once lived in Montreal, and how I'd struggled with the Québécois French. We laughed over our common difficulties with the slang street Spanish in New York. And then we were able to review his medical issues and treatment, and I could be confident that he understood.

It had never dawned on me that Mr. Mezondes might speak Spanish. I had assumed that, like most West Africans, Mr. Mezondes only spoke French in addition to his native language in Congo. And apparently it had never dawned on Mr. Mezondes that I might speak Spanish. I guess he'd assumed that most white Americans didn't speak anything but English.

"Hasta luego," he said, shaking my hand.

"*Ojalá que pasa un buen día,*" I replied, with a small surge of pride that I'd nailed the subjunctive. I knew that Mr. Mezondes would appreciate the linguistic leap that grammatical construct had entailed.

Mr. Mezondes left my office to make his appointment with the front-desk staff. Most of the Bellevue clerks were Hispanic, bilingual in Spanish and English. Mr. Mezondes—a native Congolese who spoke scant English—would have no trouble at all arranging his health care.

Now, years later, I sat with Amadou Sow from Mali in almost the same circumstance. I marveled at the ease of dialing 1800 and pressing #2 for French, though this meant we'd probably never have the opportunity to stumble on some unexpected language that we might share. A Haitian-accented voice came on and I handed the second phone line to Mr. Sow. I introduced myself and began asking about his medical history. I watched his face crease with concentration as the interpreter relayed the information to him. Within seconds of Mr. Sow's beginning his answer, the interpreter was transmitting the information about his headaches to me.

Simultaneous interpretation is a brilliant invention, but it isn't necessarily the easiest situation to navigate. Amadou Sow sat less than two feet away from me, speaking rapidly in African-accented French. His voice naturally dominated our small space. But at the same time, through the telephone at my ear, the interpreter conveyed the translation to me in soft-spoken, Haitian-accented English. The loud French and the soft English burrowed into my head at the same time, a cacophony of verbal stimuli that nearly short-circuited my brain. I had no choice but to actively block out the French in order to comprehend the English.

We'd always been taught to keep our focus on the patient, not the interpreter (whether the interpreter was a human in the room or a voice on the phone). But this was impossible during simultaneous interpretation. The only way to concentrate on the content of the English in the telephone was to tune out the patient—visually and verbally. I closed my eyes and tried to close one ear to decrease the external stimuli.

This particular patient interview was fairly straightforward. Mr. Sow had run-of-the-mill tension headaches. When I reassured him that this was not a brain tumor, that Tylenol or aspirin would suffice, he was jubilant. He pumped my hand with gratitude that he was not about to die of cancer, and then bounded out of the room, off to his weekly soccer match in Flushing Meadows. I imagined that the other Amadou Sow used to play soccer also, maybe in a league, maybe with his sons.

I started typing my note into the computer. The phone rang as I was entering the physical exam, reflecting on how different were the bodies of my two Amadou Sows. I picked up the phone and answered absentmindedly while recording the normalcy of the current Mr. Sow's muscular mass.

"Hello, Doctor." The voice was familiar enough for me to know that I'd spoken to this person before but not so familiar that I could pin it to a face.

I kept typing, now recording the normal cranial nerve functions, hoping the person would identify himself and not leave me in the awkward position of fumbling to make the connection.

"Is this Dr. Ofri?" the voice asked.

"Yes," I replied, typing in the normal patellar, Achilles, and brachioradialis reflexes. I still couldn't place the voice.

"This is the French interpreter who just assisted you with your previous patient."

The interpreter? Now I was sufficiently startled out of my workaday routine to take my hands off the keyboard and pay attention. I didn't recall ever having an interpreter call me back. In fact, I didn't recall ever having a direct conversation with an interpreter; our relationship usually ended as soon as the need for communication with a patient was over. Why would an interpreter need to talk to me? Had I committed some linguistic sin? Called him a translator instead of an interpreter? Offended Francophile sensibilities? Mangled my direct objects? Dangled my participles?

"I wanted to ask you a question, if you don't mind."

"Of course not," I said, still searching my memory.

He hesitated. Then he cleared his throat. "Doctor, what is the difference between *illness* and *disease?*"

At that I really had to sit back and pause. Not only was I being contacted by a member of the medical world with whom I'd never actually spoken directly, but I was being asked a thoughtful question, one that, as far as I could recall, had never been raised by any intern, resident, or faculty member.

"You know," I said, pushing away the keyboard, "I don't think I've ever considered this before." I stopped to think about it for a minute, twisting the phone cord into figure eights. "There is a different feel to each of these words. I know that I instinctively use *disease* and *illness* in different situations." The computer screen went blank from the inactivity, and my mind felt free to wander. I tried to come up with examples of when I'd use one word over the other, but it was hard to articulate a precise distinction to clarify to my questioner.

Was it a linguistic hairsplitting, I wondered, or was there a true difference in meaning? And perhaps this was unique to English. In Spanish, I could think of only one word that meant disease, *enfermedad.*

The interpreter told me that there was also only one word in French, *maladie,* which was why he was having so much difficulty with the two terms in English. The interpreter and I spoke more, and I found myself working through—for the first time—this interesting quirk of language. I told him that I usually used the word *disease* when talking about the biological process. I would talk about diabetes as a disease of the pancreas, a disease that could cause kidney failure, blindness, and heart attacks. But I usually used the word *illness* when I referred to the patient having the disease. I would talk about Mr. Helal's serious illness, or how Mrs. Escobar's family was dealing with her illness.

As we spoke, I could feel a distinct easing of tension in my body. The mere act of thinking and probing was a respite from the chaos of mindless tasks that usually occupied my energy. Five minutes of thoughtful discussion felt like a mini-vacation. I found myself so grateful for this interpreter who'd popped up into my day, offering this moment of relief.

A peculiar feeling remained with me after we hung up. In the nebulous void of the vast hospital machinery, I'd made a nub of a connection with a faceless, nameless voice. I'd found a brief kinship with someone who was interested in actually thinking about what we do. But with a click of the phone it had evaporated, and we were both back in our own little microscopic worlds. I didn't know his name. I didn't know where he worked or how to reach him other than to dial 1800 and press #2—but who knew how many French interpreters there were? How would I describe him to someone else, other than his having a Haitian accent and an inquisitive mind?

From then on, whenever I had a French-speaking patient and called the interpretation service, I introduced myself by name, hoping I'd find my friend again. But I didn't happen upon him.

Then, on a Thursday afternoon several weeks later, a patient from Guinea showed up in my clinic. Nobody around spoke Maninka, so I dialed 1800 and pressed #2. When I introduced myself, the voice said, "Hi, Dr. Ofri. Long time, no speak!"

After we finished with the patient, I didn't let the interpreter hang up. I said good-bye to my patient and then crammed the phone back to my ear. He introduced himself as Evans, a thirty-four-year-old man from Haiti, a real person. "How do you do it?" I wanted to know. How could a person listen in one language and speak in another at the same time, with the speaking paced two beats behind the listening?

"You either have it in you or you don't," Evans told me, confirming my suspicion that I did not. During his training, he was placed between two people who fired off phrases at him in English and in French. At first it was nearly impossible to compartmentalize his brain. He had to disengage his ear and his mouth, allowing only one narrow channel to connect them. He'd hear the phrase in French and force his mouth to speak it in English. "You can't think," he said, "you just have to do it."

I was in awe of what Evans was describing. This was an entire skill set that I did not possess, that I could not even envision myself ever acquiring. With sustained and focused effort, I can occasionally rub my belly and pat my head at the same time. This greatly impresses my children, but it is about the limit of my simultaneous abilities.

Evans told me that while he was interpreting, he found himself almost in a trance and rarely remembered what was said during the episode. Interpreters were trained to stay in a "black box," and being distant on the phone helped. It was much harder to stay in that black box when in the room with the patient.

I learned from Evans how French was structurally different from English. The questions that doctors typically piled on in list form—Do you have fever? Chills? Chest pain? Shortness of breath?—didn't work so well in French. Evans had to make a full sentence for each one, otherwise the patient would get lost.

Initials were difficult. "Doctors always say things like *HIV*," Evans said, "but I can't just translate those letters; it doesn't make any sense in French. I need to explain the whole term: *virus de l'immunodéficience humaine*. But the doctor just keeps on talking."

Evans expressed perplexity at the term *water pill*. "Why don't the doctors just say *diuretic*?" he asked me.

Hydrochlorothiazide was too much of a tongue-twister, and the word *diuretic* might not be understood. In Spanish, I always called it *pastilla de agua*—the pill that makes you produce water.

"To most patients," Evans said, "a water pill is a placebo."

Was that what my patients were thinking about the prescriptions I was giving to them?

When I told him that we typically use the term *sugar pill* to describe a placebo, he replied, "To most Haitians, a sugar pill sounds like it has something in it—actual food. But a water pill sounds like there's nothing."

Evans told me about the time he'd interpreted for a Haitian woman with breast cancer. When the cancer had been diagnosed two years earlier, the patient had said yes to all of the doctor's treatment plans but then never showed up for any appointments. Because she didn't see any visible wound on her breast, she didn't think anything was really wrong—she wasn't sick.

Two years later, she was back in the doctor's office. The cancer that could have been cured with ease had metastasized, and the doctor was crestfallen that the patient had waited so long to come back. The doctor painstakingly outlined the treatment plan—chemotherapy, hormonal therapy, possibly radiation or surgery. The patient listened politely and again said yes to everything. Then at the end she said, "Just give me some ointment for the breast. I will use the ointment and drink a special tea."

"This cancer can kill you," the doctor said, the shock and sadness in her voice evident even to Evans. "Don't you understand?"

"My breast doesn't hurt," the patient replied, "so it won't kill me. I just need ointment and a special tea."

At that point, Evans had felt compelled to intervene and talk to the doctor directly. He explained that the patient had no concept of cancer, that in Haitian culture most people could not fathom having a disease if they didn't see any actual evidence of it.

It took almost an hour, step by step, to explain about cancer and what it was and what it could do. In the end, the patient began to grasp that she could feel very sick soon, and possibly die, without treatment. Although she didn't fully comprehend the idea of a disease without any obvious signs, she began to understand that treatment might help her. She finally agreed to stay in the hospital for chemotherapy.

I hung up the phone, humbled by and envious of Evans's talent. To be fluent in two languages, to be truly bilingual, was something that I hungered for. I appreciated that I possessed enough Spanish to negotiate the basics of patient care, but I was limited to the concrete. When I ran into complex situations, as with Julia Barquero, my inability to be subtle or metaphorical or sophisticated frustrated me to no end. I didn't want to spend my entire professional life sounding like a competent third-grader, but my on-again, off-again approach to learning Spanish never advanced me much past this level. One of these days I'd have to move to a Spanish-speaking country. I didn't know how I was going to do it, but it was on the ever-growing list of things I wanted to accomplish.

∽ Chapter Six ∽

The phone rang while I was in the kitchen chopping onions for a Sunday-morning omelet. "Hello," I said, cramming the phone between my ear and my shoulder while maneuvering the squat cleaver I'd recently purchased in Chinatown. This was during my first year of medical school.

The phone line crackled slightly. "Hello, Danielle," came a voice through the static. It had a thick Middle Eastern accent, a voice I did not recognize.

"Hello?" I said tentatively, shoveling the onions onto a plate and starting on the peppers.

"How are you?" continued the voice familiarly. "I know it's early in New York, but we're just getting ready to leave for the evening and I thought I'd call to say hello."

I slowed my rate of chopping to think. It was an Israeli accent, a heavy one. Who did I know with such a clunky accent? "I'm...uh, fine," I said. "Just fine. How, uh, are you?"

"Good, good. Your mother and I have tickets to a concert to-night—Zubin Mehta is conducting—and we have to leave soon, so just a quick phone call."

Abba? The cleaver nearly slipped from my grip. This couldn't be my father. My father spoke perfect English. My father completed the *New York Times* crossword puzzles and was the house authority on spelling and grammar.

"Abba?" I said slowly. "Is that really you?" Shortly after I'd started college, my parents had moved to Israel. For my father, it was a return home after a thirty-year chapter in America—a chapter that had included his college education, teaching career, and raising two children. For my New York–born mother, this move was a new adventure, a first time living in a foreign country.

Then it hit me—my father was putting on an accent for me. I picked up the cleaver and sliced decisively through a bulbous red pepper. "That is the most pathetic Israeli accent," I said disdainfully. "*I* could probably fake it better." Hebrew had been a background language in our house, one that my father used on the

48

telephone with relatives. Occasionally when I was young he tried to speak to me in Hebrew, but it always seemed like an awkward exercise.

We talked for about ten minutes while I finished chopping vegetables, and over the course of the conversation, the accent faded—I supposed he'd grown tired of the joke—and his English went back to normal.

I hung up the phone and pulled out the eggs. I cracked them one after another, trying to perfect—with mixed success—the one-handed technique. I began to beat the eggs with a whisk while I thought about this odd conversation with my father. It occurred to me what was different about this call. Usually my mother initiated the phone calls to me; he always spoke afterward. This was the first time he'd called directly.

Odder still was that fact that my father wasn't really the impersonator type. His jokes were usually puns—lame ones at that. My hand on the whisk began to slow as a disconcerting realization dawned on me. This hadn't been a joke.

My father had an accent! An enormous humdinger of an accent. And this was the first time I'd ever heard it. I stood stock-still in my kitchen, hand frozen on the whisk as I contemplated this jarring reality: my father sounded like a foreigner.

The corollary that began to materialize was even more unsettling: I must have been unconsciously compensating during every single one of our thousands of conversations for my entire life.

I'd always thought I had such a good ear for languages and accents. Apparently not. I'd spent an entire life knowing that my father spoke unaccented English, and now I was learning that I had been utterly mistaken. It was as though someone had just informed me that I hadn't grown up with a black mutt from the ASPCA, or that my first-grade teacher hadn't been named Ms. Zive, or that our downstairs bathroom hadn't been lined with Peter Max wallpaper and our kitchen hadn't been painted avocado green. The "facts" of my childhood were suddenly being brusquely reordered.

It was only this one time, when his voice came to me out of context—an unexpected phone call without the preparation of talking to my mother first—that I suddenly heard the accent. And as I'd become involved in the conversation, the accent had melted away, receding as my brain quietly massaged things into the way I evidently expected them to be.

-----⊗∞⊗-----

Whenever I took stock of my efforts to learn Spanish and communicate with my patients, I often thought back to this freakish phone call that occurred during medical school. Beyond making me aware of how perception often bore only a tenuous connection to reality, it drove home the point of how ferociously difficult it was to acquire a second language in adulthood. Despite three decades of full immersion in a language, the accent could still be there.

Even so, I realized that I'd probably never equal my father's achievement. I could never envision attending college in my second language, teaching twenty-five years of high-school math in my second language, marrying someone who didn't speak my native language, raising my children in a language that was not my mother tongue, much less doing the crossword puzzle in a foreign language. My father told me that he could think and even dream in both languages, though sometimes his hand was momentarily confused when it hit the page as to whether to move left to right or right to left. I was in awe of this fluidity, especially because I knew that his exposure to English as a child had been limited to the fifth-grade grammar lessons enforced by the British Mandate that controlled Palestine at the time. When he arrived in America at the age of twenty-three, he was far more comfortable in Arabic than in English, yet he enrolled in college nevertheless.

I sweated over my Spanish—beginning in my internship year with a one-week crash course in Guatemala—knowing that I needed it for survival, knowing that it was unlikely that I'd ever navigate it smoothly. By now I'd reached a precarious middle ground in which I spoke well enough to carry on a conversation, well enough for my Hispanic patients to assume they could talk to me in Spanish. But I lacked the agility to field unexpected linguistic turns. What I could say, I could say well—but beyond that circumscribed field of comfort, I was at a loss. I had a fluency, but I was not fluent, and that could be a dangerous state of affairs.

It was a rainy Wednesday when Señora Estrella pulled a plastic zip-lock bag from her purse and plunked it dramatically on my desk—exhibit A. Inside was a drinking glass.

Nilda Estrella had knocked on my door fifteen minutes earlier, her clothes wet and windswept from the storm. She didn't have an appointment, but she needed to talk with me. It was urgent, but it wouldn't take long. "*Un ratito,*" she'd said. Only a minute. She undid her rain bonnet, wiping off the drops that had slithered underneath. Her hair was thick and black, with a prominent tuft of white in front. She settled her short square frame in the chair and leaned forward on the edge of my desk with an intense bearing.

I knew that Señora Estrella had a grown daughter who'd been diagnosed with a glioblastoma—a brain tumor—a few years back. She'd had surgery, radiation, and chemotherapy, and went into remission. But the tumor had returned, though I wasn't sure exactly where things stood right now. I geared up for the verbal onslaught.

Compared with the more deliberately articulated Spanish of the Mexican, Colombian, and Argentine patients, the Spanish of the Dominicans and Puerto Ricans was like a tsunami of pebble-strewn water. The words rattled and flew, with barely a space for breath. L's, r's, and other extraneous letters were casually dropped like excess baggage. Unnecessary words, such as pronouns and articles, were shrugged off with insouciance. Slang terms peppered the speech, alternating with Spanglish, local dialects, and frank neologisms. All of which stymied my by-the-book Spanish, learned from ever patient, slowly speaking Mexican and Guatemalan teachers.

Every visit with Señora Estrella for the past three years had been permeated by an undercurrent of anxiety about her daughter. I expected today to be the same and so I set my mind toward thinking about cancer and the fright of losing a child.

Before I knew it, however, I was lost in a verbal torrent about juicers. Organic juicers! Señora Estrella's Spanish gushed forth with something about how the home attendant—apparently the daughter now needed a home attendant—had made juice with carrots, pears, and parsley, or maybe it was apples, beets, and celery. The juice was made every day, but the particular juice in question was from last week, or maybe it was two weeks ago. After drinking the juice, Señora Estrella had felt a little nauseated and had pains in her kidneys. And her daughter had a headache and tingling in her hands. Or maybe it was the daughter with the kidney pains and the mother with the tingling. But the daughter had also been feeling these symptoms since her last radiation treatment, so maybe it wasn't from the juice.

Señora Estrella kept up her avalanche of a monologue. Her son was coming in from Santo Domingo to live with them, and the apartment was too small. Her husband wasn't working now, or maybe he was working now but hadn't been working before. Or maybe it was the son who hadn't been working but was now working. The son and the husband didn't get along, or maybe they used to not get along but now they did, or now they didn't, or wouldn't, or couldn't, or shouldn't.

Sometimes they didn't use the celery, or maybe it was the parsley, because one of them was supposed to improve your immune system and one was supposed to protect you from radiation. After finishing radiation the daughter underwent an MRI, or maybe it was a CT scan, and based on that they would soon hear from the oncologist about what treatment would be next. But the home attendant didn't have any symptoms, or maybe she did have symptoms, but she didn't drink the juice, or maybe she did drink the juice, or maybe she drank it but on a different day. But they had the juice every day, and sometimes they used red cabbage instead of red beets, because something about the red pigment was supposed to help ward off cancer.

My head spun as I floundered in her convoluted story. Should I pause to translate the more complicated words into English? I wondered. But then I'd risk falling behind in the complex tale. Or should I just follow the flow as best I could in order to extract the gestalt, then clarify details afterward?

I struggled to keep track of which thread of the story was going to turn out to be the critical one—the juicer? the brain tumor? the family dynamics? Which one would I have to hang on to in order to diagnose and treat whatever the concluding issue turned out to be? It was like being on a rubber raft bumping down rapids, trying to grab at branches poking out from trees on the shore in an attempt to create a semblance of a linear journey.

And that was when Señora Estrella abruptly ceased her commentary, pulled out the zip-lock bag, and plopped it on my desk as though it were the pinnacle of the story. She unzipped the plastic bag and eased out the cup. She pushed the cup toward me and then folded her arms, evidently waiting for the obvious diagnostic pronouncement that would clinch the thesis of her argument.

It was an ordinary empty drinking glass—unremarkable, except that it seemed an odd thing to be carrying in one's purse. I picked up the cup and twisted it in the air, peering from all angles at this strange, tangible evidence that I was hoping would clarify the serpentine saga that had just been presented to me. Inside the cup, lining the bottom, was a faint chalky white coating that flaked like old paint. Señora Estrella nodded like a barrister when she saw my gaze rest on the eggshell layer.

This was the first stretch of silence in our entire encounter, and suddenly I could breathe. My brain could actually think without having to struggle to stay above water. And now that it could think, it had no idea what to make of all this.

I began asking questions in order to tease the main story out of the earlier morass. I stuck with simple yes-or-no questions so that I could align the facts without getting too lost. Slowly I put the picture together, about how the home attendant had made the juice last week, and that both Señora Estrella and the daughter had felt sick, but that they had different symptoms, though both already felt better now. But the glass, on that day only, was left with this white residue, and Señora Estrella wanted me to send it to our laboratory for analysis to figure out what had endangered her daughter's precarious health.

I called the lab in our hospital and the technician laughed derisively at me when I asked how to submit a drinking cup for analysis.

I hung up the phone and stared dumbly at the white layer. Maybe it was calcium? Maybe it was some other mineral in the water or the vegetables? I did a quick search on the Internet and found some reports about fibrous material that could build up in the juicer, and perhaps be a nidus for bacterial growth. Señora Estrella was not satisfied with my conjectures, however, and demanded that I do something with the flaky white residue at the bottom of her cup.

By now nearly thirty minutes had elapsed, and I was worn out from her story—plus my other patients were piling up in the waiting room. I suggested that she take the cup to the poison control center and see if they would analyze it. She pursed her lips and contemplated me from hooded eyes. I could see that this did not constitute a sufficient response. Señora Estrella wasn't going to leave my office until I did something concrete.

I settled on some blood tests, even though I didn't think she needed any. Blood tests were relatively harmless, not too expensive, and might offer a reasonable placebo effect. I was usually a stickler about not doing any tests unless absolutely necessary, but it was obvious that I wasn't going to resolve this mess without giving Señora Estrella something solid. At this point, if I got her out of my office without ordering laparoscopic surgery, I'd consider it a success.

All in all, it was an entirely unsatisfying experience for both of us. I wondered if things would have worked out better if I had used an interpreter. Would a clearer understanding of her initial story have decreased my level of frustration and allowed me to be a more compassionate listener? Or would it have expanded a merely frustrating thirty-minute encounter into a painfully arduous sixty-minute ordeal?

After Señora Estrella closed the door behind her and I unkinked my stiff neck, I reached up and pulled one of my Spanish textbooks off the shelf. It was filled with page after page of comprehension exercises, conjugation charts, vocabulary lists, grammatical rules, and idiom definitions. The sheer volume and complexity was daunting. What made me think I could possibly master a second language at this stage in life? What sort of delusion was I laboring under that I could actually practice medicine in a foreign language? Was this what my father had felt when he walked into a university lecture hall for the first time?

And yet, here I was—a doctor in Bellevue Hospital, where most patients spoke Spanish. Either I was going to spend the majority of my waking hours with a translator-phone in my hand, or I was going to figure out how to speak Spanish. Could it really be any harder than the biochemistry I'd learned for the MCATs back in college? As I gazed at the fourteen possible tenses for each verb—tenses that I probably couldn't even name or define in English—I concluded that it probably *was* harder than biochemistry. After all, the pentose phosphate shunt just had to be memorized with brute force and recited for the exam; then it could be forgotten. The *pluscuamperfecto,* however, had to be painstakingly teased out—like Señora Estrella's story—and then stitched back into my speech and thought. Not to mention that *pluscuamperfecto* could exist in the indicative mode or the subjunctive mode—modes we barely considered in English but which were crucial in Spanish.

Mr. Mezondes seemed to have figured it out. If a French-speaking African could navigate English-speaking America with only the Spanish he'd learned in Congo, then certainly I should be able to manage here in New York City. If Dr. Chan could negotiate Medicaid and the INS based on Fukienese Shakespeare classes in the 1950s, then I could probably extricate a bit more leverage from my language skills.

There was a lot of verbiage out there in the great wide world of Bellevue and beyond, and if I wanted any hope of maneuvering my way through cancer treatments, organic juicers, and complex patient expectations, I'd better get cracking. I tucked the Spanish book into my bag to bring home that night. Forget the gym—I needed to be bench-pressing the pluperfect.

Two months later, I still hadn't heard any follow-up about the juicer mystery. Señora Estrella's blood tests had been, as I'd expected, perfectly normal. If anything further had gone wrong, I would surely have heard about it. Now I was sitting in my office with Wilamena Ortiz. A diminutive, energetic woman with practical haircuts and no-nonsense shoes, she was one of my healthy patients. Sometimes her arthritis acted up, but that never stopped her from walking eight laps around the block every day. Occasionally she had bronchitis, but mostly we just talked about ways to keep healthy. These were the fun visits that I genuinely enjoyed: no impending death or doom, no chronic debilitating illnesses. We got to focus on the preventive measures like Pap tests, mammograms, exercise, and vaccines—things that often got shunted to the side when a patient had multiple severe diseases.

The other reason that I enjoyed our visits was that Wilamena Ortiz was from Peru. Peruvian Spanish was clear and steady. Each word was fully articulated, and every letter was pronounced—crucial elements for a midlevel Spanish speaker like me. Visits with Señora Ortiz left me with the heady feeling that I had truly mastered the language, since I could understand just about every word she said. I felt confident that almost nothing was shortchanged in our encounter and that, unlike the case with Señora Estrella, language was not an impediment to good medical care.

Señora Ortiz was here for an annual checkup and had no medical concerns to report, so I asked her a general question about how things were going at home. She replied that she was actually under quite a bit of stress these days, especially regarding her older daughter. She started telling me a complicated story about her daughter's boyfriend, their young child, the discord in their relationship, how the daughter was starting to rely on her mother more but that the two of them were beginning to fight.

Her voice became more staccato as she grew emotional, talking about the pain that her daughter's troubles were causing her. Her mild eyes grew taut, and her words began to run together, the final consonants of one word bumping up against the following word.

The crisp Peruvian articulation began to break down. I found that I was beginning to miss a word here and there, and I worried that I might lose the thread of her increasingly complex story. I cocked my head closer to her, as though absorbing more of her voice might help me understand more. Señora Ortiz was now biting her lip to hold back tears, and her speech became ragged as she told me that she was concerned that her daughter might be the victim of abuse by her boyfriend.

I pulled the box of tissues closer to us, and I reached out for Señora Ortiz's hand. She swallowed hard, but the tears began to flow anyway. Now her voice was savaged by emotion, and I could feel my grasp of her Spanish slipping away.

I felt as though I'd been thrust into the same precarious situation I'd been in with Señora Estrella. Should I let her know that I was losing track of her story? Should I stop and call an interpreter? But that would be too disruptive, obviously, at such an emotional moment. I longed for someone like Evans lodged in my auditory cortex, catching the foreign-language words before they burrowed in, instantly converting them to English, maintaining the rhythm, tone, prosody, idioms, and emotional nuances so that I could possess a confident grip on the myriad denotations and connotations of Señora Ortiz's story.

Lacking that, I could only narrow my eyes and focus my brain intently on her rocky torrent. Señora Ortiz grabbed my hand in both of hers and pulled me closer. From her increasingly muddled speech I discerned that she herself had been abused when she was younger, and now she was afraid that her daughter was ending up in the same situation.

Now it was my turn to be anxious. This was getting serious and I had to be sure that I understood, yet I felt that I couldn't stop her in the middle. Bits and pieces came flying now: her difficult life in Peru with her first husband, how she'd left with three children and come to America, how she'd survived with no English and no money, how she'd sacrificed to give her children a better life, but now it seemed that her daughter was falling into the same trap that she had, and she was powerless to stop it.

I knew that I was missing some details and certainly many of the nuances, but she hung on to me while she spoke, and I hung on to her story as it unfolded. I hoped that I was getting the gist of it, but I couldn't be entirely sure.

And then, finally, we arrived at the other shore: Señora Ortiz had finished her story. Her terror seeped into silence as we both took deep breaths. The grip of our hands loosened and a cathartic calm tentatively settled in the room.

Her exhausted Spanish eased its way back to its normal pitch and clarity as we talked quietly about options for handling her situation: consulting a therapist, talking to her priest, confiding in friends. I gave her the phone number of a domestic-violence hotline, as well as the number of our social worker. We lamented, though, the limited steps she could take with respect to her daughter's life. There was almost nothing, it seemed, to compare to the pain of watching one's child—at any age—get hurt. I thought about my two young children and the depth of effort Benjy and I were investing to give them a safe, happy environment enriched with books, music lessons, museums, concerts, whole wheat pasta, SPF 50 sunscreen, safety-approved car seats, accredited day care. These ramparts of childhood we were so busy erecting suddenly appeared friable as Señora Ortiz spoke. No matter how many variables of our children's lives we sought to control, our ability to protect them would gradually crumble as they grew up.

We walked to the door together and bade each other farewell. As with Señora Estrella, I second-guessed myself: should I have obtained an interpreter when I began to lose my grasp of the story? Perhaps I'd missed important information that would somehow affect her health and safety. But if an interpreter had been the go-between, would she have spoken as freely about her painful memories? Was it more crucial that I simply remained there, allowing her to unload her story? Was I practicing medicine with overly flawed tools?

I often thought about what my father's first day of teaching must have been like—standing in front of a class of skeptical tenth-graders with his medium grasp of English and an accent heavy enough to sink a freighter. Here I was in a similar situation, attempting a professional interaction despite blatant conjugational sins, an intransigent inability to conceptualize male versus female nouns, an utter indifference to direct versus indirect objects, and the occasional horrendous malapropism (like the time I'd asked a patient *¿Cúantos anos tiene?* rather than *¿Cúantos años tiene?*

She was polite enough not to point out that I'd just asked her how many anuses she had rather than how old she was). Yet whenever I offered my patients a choice, they overwhelmingly preferred direct communication—even if somewhat flawed—to the unnatural stiffness of an interposed interpreter, no matter how perfect the translation.

For me, learning Spanish was a never-ending and forever frustrating, humbling process. Full mastery always seemed just out of reach.

∾ Chapter Seven ∾

Azad Aptekin was thirty years old. Slightly built, fair-skinned, with thinning, receding hair, he wore neat khaki pants and a casual button-down shirt. His shoes were comfortable black leather. Unlike many foreigners, his clothes were distinctly American, sort of a relaxed-preppy look. His features were dark, eyes cautious, finely chiseled in his smooth, oval face. My first reaction, even before guessing what country he was from—which I couldn't quite place from his appearance—was that he was probably gay. I gave myself a mental kick in the shins for letting this be my first thought, but that was what came to me on that Monday afternoon at one.

We introduced ourselves, and he told me he was from Turkey. He had grown up in Konya, and when I told him that I'd visited that city, his face lit up. Konya was the home of the famous Sufi poet Rumi and has historically been a spiritual, mystical place. Though it had been two decades since I'd visited, I had a pristine recollection of entering the famous mosque, draping my shorts and T-shirt with heavy, musty shawls before crossing the threshold.

As Mr. Aptekin and I spoke, I wondered why I had been so immediately convinced that he was gay. Nothing in our conversation alluded to that, and I decided that I wouldn't specifically ask unless it seemed relevant. Mr. Aptekin told me his story, that he'd been involved in politics as a student in Turkey and had become a human rights activist. Without elaborating much, he told me that he'd been arrested, beaten, and sexually assaulted—sadly, the standard SOT story. He eventually left Turkey, lived in Europe, then in 2001 came to the United States. He'd studied finance in Boston, earning an MBA. He'd worked in the banking industry in Chicago for a while but found the frenetic pace of work unsettling. Now he did real estate in New York, and the independence agreed with him. "If it's a good day, I go out and work. If it's a bad day, I'm able to stay home."

In the Social History part of the medical interview, I made the requisite inquiries about toxic habits, but he'd never smoked, drunk alcohol, or used any drugs. He smiled and said, "I grew up

in a very conservative Muslim family; none of that *ever* happened."
Then I asked the standard questions about whether he was married
(no), currently sexually active (no), had been sexually active in the
past (yes). When I delved further, Mr. Aptekin replied that he'd had
some boyfriends in the past, but none now.

My instinct had been correct. I wondered whether he might
have been singled out for arrest and torture in Turkey because of
his sexual orientation, but I couldn't think of a comfortable way to
ask, at least at this moment. I could only imagine that for someone
growing up in a conservative Muslim family in the most conservative city of Konya, it would be extremely difficult to be homo-
sexual.

"Are you in touch with your family?" I finally asked.

"I call them," Mr. Aptekin said, "but the conversations are
brief. They just want to know when I am getting married."

I raised my eyebrows and he returned my gaze. After a pause I
asked quietly, "Could you ever tell them?"

"Never," he said flatly, straightening the cuff on his left sleeve,
then glancing at the face of his silver watch. "It's beyond their comprehension. It would bring such shame on them in the community;
it would ruin their lives. I couldn't do that to them."

"How about your siblings?" Mr. Aptekin had told me he was
one of eleven children, almost all of whom were living in Europe
or America.

"I've never told them and we never discuss it."

"Do you think they know? After all, they're living in the
West..."

"I'm sure some of them have figured it out." He hung his head
low, and for a moment I thought he might cry. "But we never mention it. We all know that it would devastate my parents, so it stays
under the table."

This elaborate cloak of secrecy among eleven siblings on three
continents over years and years seemed untenable to me. "How
long can you live like this?" I asked.

"Until my parents die," he replied matter-of-factly. He shrugged,
but there was a pained finality in his voice.

We were silent for a few minutes. Mr. Aptekin's gaze traveled slowly around the room, not settling on anything. "How old are they?" I asked gingerly.

"In their seventies," he said. "So..." His last word hung in the air, like an acrid aftertaste.

I wondered about the intricacies of Azad Aptekin's life. He was thirty years old, unable to be open about his life with anyone in his family. I imagined he'd be angry, yet he seemed most concerned with sparing his parents any pain or shame. Where did he find it within himself to protect them? Since his arrest and torture in Turkey, he'd suffered from depression, anxiety, and insomnia. How could this ever resolve if he couldn't derive comfort from his family?

"Are you in any danger?" I asked.

"Not from my immediate family," he said in a manner that suggested he didn't take this for granted, "but there are relatives who would kill me, I am sure." He leaned forward, thrusting his forearms against his thighs. His eyes narrowed, and rancor palpably agitated his voice. "You've heard about 'honor killings,' yes? Well, they'd do the same to people like me, if they knew. I can't ever go back to Turkey."

Mr. Aptekin had stopped both the therapy and the antidepressant medications that his psychiatrist had initially recommended. "I'm not sick," he said sharply, running a finger along the crease of his pants. "I don't like depending on anyone or anything." His head sank low again and remained there for the rest of our visit.

Mr. Aptekin struck me as almost more disillusioned, and far sadder, than Samuel Nwanko. Samuel's life had clearly been irreparably damaged, yet he hadn't seemed embittered; somehow he was able to focus on moving forward.

But Azad Aptekin seemed trapped. Despite escaping the country of his torture, he remained ensnared in the web of his prior existence, like a freed slave who never feels fully free—or never actually is free. Perhaps the death of his parents would release him from the prison that he carried with him across the ocean. But what a depressing way to view liberation.

Or perhaps nothing would change after his parents died. Perhaps the prison bars had become internalized—ossified and incorporated into his very marrow, rendering him incapable of being himself even after his parents and his Turkish jailers ceased to exist.

By midafternoon on Mondays, I was always eager to return to the ordinary deadliness of renal failure, cirrhosis, myocardial infarctions, pneumonia, and diabetic complications. At least there were prescriptions that could be written and treatment plans to dispense. There was even the occasional hope of cure.

I'd never heard of Jean-Baptiste Lully. Don't worry, my teacher said, no one's ever heard of him unless they've used the Suzuki books. The *Gavotte* that was Lully's great contribution to the Suzuki pedagogy was a Slavic-sounding dance with deep-throated rhythms that seem particularly suited to the cello. The piece wasn't as challenging as some of the others we'd worked on, but the syncopations and bowing were good exercises. I tried to play the *Gavotte* at least once during my evening practice sessions, like a daily vitamin, but I couldn't start my practice until the kids had taken their baths, gotten into their pajamas, brushed their teeth, and had their stories read to them. When I first began the cello, I had fantasies of serenading Naava and Noah to sleep. But early attempts at stringed instruments are notoriously squawky. Every night I diligently played the A, D, G, and C strings—the only thing I could do—until finally Naava piped up from bed, "Do you know any other notes?"

Tonight I was practicing in my bedroom, since its walls did not abut the neighbors' apartments and I could spare them the nightly drone. I was midway through the *Gavotte* when Naava tiptoed into my brightly lit room. She surreptitiously climbed into my bed, and I pretended not to notice. During a half-note rest on the second page I said, "Two minutes only," and she responded by pulling the quilt more snugly around her shoulders. I pressed on with the rest of the piece, which reaches a fortissimo finale. I crashed the last note with as much oomph as possible, racing the bow across the strings with a dramatic flourish as my teacher had instructed.

The last note was still reverberating as I glanced toward the bed. Naava was sound asleep, snoring softly, oblivious to my music, to my concertizing efforts as well as to my mistakes. I was grateful for such a tolerant audience.

I put away the cello, then scooped Naava in my arms. Her string bean of a body offered no resistance and slumped comfortably into mine. As I carried her back to her room, I was enveloped in the heady scent of childhood, body and hair still redolent of talcum powder even though we were long past that stage. I slid Naava into her bed, then spied Noah's two stuffed iguana brothers on the floor under a pile of books. I rescued Elliot Iguanadon and Eliezer Iguanadon from the crush and tucked them in the crook of Noah's arm before easing the bedroom door shut.

I clicked open my laptop, just for a minute, to check e-mail—I'd sworn to get to bed earlier—but I was curious about Lully, wondering who this person was whose music I was mangling more than three hundred years after he'd composed it. I'll only take a moment, I promised myself, but then one interesting tidbit led to another. An hour later, I was still reading about Jean-Baptiste Lully, the son of a miller in a small French village, uneducated, looking forward to a life of grinding grain. But like the force of the river that relentlessly drove the waterwheel of the family mill, his musical talent surged to the surface and he was propelled into the bright orbit of Parisian society. Lully's artistic proclivity was unstoppable, and he eventually found his way into the court of Louis XIV. He composed and performed for the king, and collaborated with Molière. Lully was wildly popular, a fixture of the cultural scene. He was also bisexual, flaunting his affairs with men and women alike.

I paused for a moment, contemplating the openness with which Jean-Baptiste Lully was able to conduct his life three centuries ago compared with the constricted existence of Azad Aptekin.

Lully bounced from one meteoric scandal to another, always managing to resurrect himself due to his prodigious musical talent. His eventual demise turned out to be a result of his musical life, though, not his libertine excesses. Before the advent of short batons, conductors used long wooden staffs to beat time on the floor. During one concert, Lully slammed his toe while conducting. A gangrenous abscess developed and the doctors recommended amputation of the toe. Lully refused—some said out of vanity—and gangrene disseminated rapidly, leading to his death at age fifty-five.

Lully lives on, mainly in the legions of Suzuki students who plod through his *Gavotte,* wholly unaware, I was sure, of both his sexual exuberance and his death by occupational hazard.

I closed the laptop, reflexively muffling the metallic click because the kids were sleeping, though I realized this was ridiculous since Naava had managed to fall asleep two feet from a booming cello. I climbed into bed, envious of the ease and depth of my children's repose, of their ability to plunge so ardently into untroubled slumber. Whenever I attempted to sleep, the closing of my eyes was simply the cue for the reels of my daytime worries to roll for a rebroadcast. Against a now tenebrous background, replays of Azad Aptekin's corrosive internal pain, Samuel Nwanko's scarred face, Julia Barquero's doomed heart, and now Jean-Baptiste Lully's fatal gangrenous toe cycled until I eventually sank into a fitful sleep.

Part Two

The water shimmered in the sunlight, casting diamondlike sparkles. The heat was brutal—hot enough for the leaves on the trees to wilt. Brookfield River rippled temptingly, and the other teenagers bobbed in and out with drenched excitement. It was December 6, a week before high-school graduation, a week before summer vacation. The verdant New Zealand landscape rolled for miles beyond the river, the green hazy in the languorous heat.

Jade Collier sat in the front passenger seat of the beat-up green Vauxhall that was pulled up to the edge of the river. She eyed the cool, glistening water, watching her friends swim. Gushes of water lapped over the edge, dousing the riverbank's knot of weeds and rushes. She chided herself for forgetting her bathing suit. But this outing hadn't been planned; at the last minute, she and her friends had cut out of Bible study. They'd changed into their best hippie clothes, piled into the Vauxhall, and drove the six miles from Napier to Brookfield River, where now the water beckoned achingly. Water had always been a magnet for Jade and her twin sister, Judith. As young children, they used to take swims in the cows' water troughs on the family farm. Anywhere there was water, Jade needed to be in it. If it weren't for the fact that she was wearing her favorite T-shirt—white with a bold red-patterned peace sign—she would have jumped in with her clothes on.

The old Collier dairy farm was an hour away—a lifetime away—in the village of Purtorino. Purtorino was considered a bigger village because it boasted a pub and two auto shops in addition to the standard village store. The village center sported exactly four houses—one for the family that owned the pub, one for the family that owned the store, and one for each family that owned an auto shop. There were three more houses near the school—and that was the extent of the downtown. The rest of the area was made up of thousand-acre farms spread out through the vast countryside.

At three hundred acres, the Collier farm was smaller than most, but it seemed enormous to Jade, Judith, and their older sisters, Katy and Naomi. They grew up with the animals, helping to feed the

calves, milking the young ones that weren't ready for the mecha-
nized milkers. After school, they climbed into the henhouse to feed
the squawking *chooks*.

Life on the farm came to a screeching halt when Jade's father
died of liver cancer. At age thirteen, Jade and her twin sister were
sent off to boarding school in Napier, a bustling city of forty-five
thousand people. Their mother attempted to lease the farm, share
the farm, rent parts of it, but none of these plans succeeded. After
two years, she gave up, sold the farm, and joined the girls in Napier.
She pulled the girls out of boarding school, and they started life
again together as a family, but absent a father.

In retrospect, Jade could identify these upheavals as the source
of her teenage anger—an anger that was unfocused, unresolved,
and unremitting. Her mother wasn't the type of person who aired
or analyzed difficult emotions. Her marriage had been an unhappy,
uncommunicative one—its dissolution by death a disagreeable mix
of grief, guilt, and relief. She tended to sulk, and in that vacuum the
Collier girls ran wild.

In Napier, Jade and Judith hooked up with the Hawke's Bay
Hippies. Though there was plenty of partying, smoking, beer
drinking, hitchhiking, and cutting out of school and church, it was
still relatively tame. Hard drugs hadn't yet made an appearance in
small-town New Zealand of the 1970s. Rebellion was in the form
of miniskirts and sneaking out of Bible study. The teenagers dressed
and acted like hippies—sporting peace signs and beads—even
though no one had ever so much as laid eyes on an actual hippie.

Both Judith and Jade had been accepted into nursing school,
following in Katy's footsteps. While the twins were evading Bible
study and loitering at Brookfield River on that Sunday, Katy was
on duty at the Napier hospital.

The sultry, sticky interior of the Vauxhall was oppressive, and
the sight of everyone else frolicking in the water made it even more
so. Maybe the water wouldn't really harm the shirt, Jade considered. The colors probably wouldn't run. But what if it got caught on
a branch? What if it got stained from the reeds? What if it shrunk?

Finally she succumbed. "Ah, heck," she muttered, and then

dashed out of the car. It was only four steps to the water's edge. She took it running, and dove cleanly into the shimmering water. She turned her head to the left as she dove in, noticing a log that her body had neatly cleared. The delicious coolness of the water sheathed her body in relief.

And then she heard a soft ping. That was it, just a soft, low-pitched ping.

A humming rose in her ears and Jade found herself in a V position under the water, facing downward. She pulled herself up, or at least did what she thought was pulling herself up, but all that resulted from her efforts was a faint waggling of her hands. She jerked her body upward more forcefully, or at least that's what her mind commanded. But nothing happened. It was then that Jade realized that she couldn't move, that she was trapped underwater, paralyzed.

She was fully conscious, and remained oddly calm. Her only thought was a very rational *I do hope somebody gets me out soon.* She knew she had to hold her breath, but having spent the last few years competing with her sisters as to who could stay underwater the longest, she had faith in her lungs. Her body remained frozen underwater while she held her breath, counting slowly. The other swimmers kept on swimming; the Hawke's Bay Hippies noticed nothing amiss.

It is often said that there is a certain extrasensory connection between twins. Judith, who was on the shore, knew right away that something was wrong. She began screaming, the type of bone-shattering scream that commands immediate attention. Her words were choked but her friends followed her frenzied gestures toward the river. Three teenagers plunged into the waist-deep water and hauled her twin sister out. It had been about two minutes.

At first they stretched Jade out on the bank, thinking she'd gotten water in her lungs and just needed a few moments to recover. They leaned over her limp, wet body, arguing about how best to extract water from the lungs. Jade was conscious but had only a fuzzy awareness of what has happening. All she knew was that she couldn't feel her stomach. She demanded that someone pour water on her stomach. One of the boys complied, hustling a bucket of river water and dumping it haphazardly onto her midsection.

After a few minutes, it became evident that the situation was more serious than they'd thought. Someone shouted that they had to get her to the hospital—there was no phone nearby to call an ambulance. The teenagers crammed their arms under her body and lifted her into the green Vauxhall. They tried headfirst, then feet-first, but the ancient sedan couldn't fit the length of Jade's body. With no knowledge of how paramedics typically immobilized body and neck on a flat board, the Hawke's Bay Hippies bent Jade's body into a sitting position and squeezed her into the back seat. They piled into the car to support her—six in all—and gunned the engine, racing toward the hospital.

The Vauxhall was immediately pulled over by the cops for speeding. Urgent, agitated voices heaped one on top of another, competing to describe the accident. Somehow through the verbal cacophony they managed to convey the medical urgency. The police turned on their siren and led the way, speeding down the road to the hospital.

In the emergency room that day, Katy Collier was the admitting nurse. By constitution, Katy was a coolheaded person. Nothing rattled her, and when her little sister was extracted from the carful of panting teenagers, she retained her professional demeanor.

It was this preternatural composure that kept Jade from panicking. *If Katy is calm,* she thought as she was being loaded onto a stretcher, *everything will be all right.* Her only panic arose when another nurse pulled out a scissor and began slicing open her clothing. "No," Jade screamed. She would not let them cut her precious peace shirt. "No," she screamed again, and began fighting off the nurse. But her body remained immobile. There was no fighting that could be done.

———

No one ever said, "You're never going to walk again"—or if someone did, Jade blocked it out. Katy seemed to believe that Jade would heal, and if Katy believed it, then Jade did too. Shortly after the accident, Jade was transferred from North Island to South

Island—the other half of New Zealand—where the hospital had a specialized rehab unit for spinal injury.

In the first few weeks at the rehab, Jade was flat on her back, unable to do anything. Therapists rotated and manipulated her limbs to maintain flexibility, but it was as though they were merely pantomiming in the air. All of her body felt removed, distant, almost nonexistent. While lying flat, Jade spent hours visualizing how she would walk out of the plane, triumphantly returning home to North Island. She chose and discarded endless combinations of clothes, determined to pick the exact right outfit for a walking debut. In the end she settled on brown suede boots, a suede jacket with fringes, and a matching purse—also brown suede, also fringed. Though she was fully aware that her legs did not work, somehow that didn't translate to her not ever walking again. She assumed that she'd be walking within a year.

Christmas Day came three weeks after the accident. Jade had never been alone on Christmas, and now she was far from her family, isolated in a strange place, in a strange life. The hospital cooked a version of Christmas dinner, but it was a sad imitation. It was cold when it arrived at her bedside—the ham limp, the mashed potatoes congealed, the stuffing dry. And then someone had to spoon it to into her mouth, bit by flavorless bit.

The spinal-injury ward housed fifteen patients; Jade was the youngest, and the only girl. The others, in their twenties, were far more worldly. They coached Jade as she began the grueling process of regaining strength in her lax limbs. Each muscle had to be coaxed painfully and arduously, seemingly one fiber at a time. Slowly, her fingers began to respond, then her hands—holding a book so that she could read became her most fervent goal.

Although one might expect a ward full of young people with severed spinal cords to be a dreary place, in fact, the ward had a summer-camp atmosphere—teenagers on their own, no parents, only young nurses as their "counselors." The nurses frequently took patients on trips, often to movies, parties. With the help of able-bodied visitors, water balloons could be lobbed over the balconies, pillows could be brandished like shields, and generalized mayhem could be engendered.

By the end of the five months, Jade's arms allowed her to propel herself a few feet in a manual wheelchair. The time had come to return home to North Island, but she would not be stepping out of a plane in her brown suede, fringed hippie outfit. She would be in a wheelchair, and before she could return to her home, she first had to transfer back to the Napier hospital for several days.

The summer camp was over, and Jade was plunged into an atmosphere that lacked any of the sensitivity of the spinal-cord-injury unit. An aide wheeled Jade to the shower one day and was not attentive to the dimensions of the chair, plowing into an elderly woman in the hallway. The woman threw Jade a how-dare-you look, then walked away, shaking her head in disgust before Jade could even explain.

Two days later Jade was wheeled in a commode chair, but the aide had neglected to attach the crucial bottom tray. Jade had limited bladder and bowel control and was mortified to discover that she was leaving a trail down the hall, just like the horses in Purtorino.

She was finally discharged from the local hospital, five months after cutting out of Bible class on that sunny afternoon. Jade was home, but not ready for the logistics of the real world. Though she wasn't technically incontinent, she had less than a minute's grace period after the realization that she had to go. This simply would not do for a social outing, so she declined every invitation, inventing various and sundry excuses. This, along with her mother's over-protectiveness, served to keep her cloistered for the better part of a year. It was also the year that the reality of the permanence of her paralysis set in. She'd still been holding on to the hope that her spine might heal and that she would be able to walk. But facing the four walls of her house, day in and day out, gradually extinguished that hope.

Jade's restive teenage anger surfaced, and she decided that she had to take her life in her own hands. Armed with a portable loo and the resolve that she'd tell people that they'd simply have to avert their eyes during this momentary emergency, she took a part-time job in an office. This led to a full-time job and finally to a car that gave her the freedom to act out just like she used to do.

Jade returned to partying, drinking, smoking. She leapfrogged through serial short-term boyfriends, always being the first to break it off. And then one day, as Jade recalled it, "God spoke to me." It was a low but audible voice in her head, and it told her that she needed to move to Australia. Jade hadn't been that active with the church, but she had no doubt that it was the voice of God, and that if she didn't listen, she'd regret it.

She pulled out a map of Australia and selected Brisbane, a city on the southeast coast known for its mild winters. If she was going to strike out on her own, risk everything she had, she might as well do it in pleasant weather.

With little more than the address of a halfway house for the disabled, Jade flew herself to Brisbane and talked her way into a room. Her next stop was the local pub. Networking was easy over a few pints, and she quickly made friends and found herself an office job. For more than a decade, she relished the bustling life of this city that was bisected by the snaking Brisbane River. She had several serious boyfriends, relationships that now lasted years rather than weeks. It was with Jordon that she first contemplated marriage. They planned to move to Africa together, to stake out an even more adventurous life. She didn't know how wheelchair-amenable the jungles of Africa might be, but she was willing to take her chances. If something wasn't accessible, she'd figure out a way to make it so.

Just before the Africa trip, she paid a visit to Katy, who was now living in Brooklyn, New York, and God spoke to her for the second time, again with regard to travel plans. This time it was a stern warning—not to go to Africa. The words were plain and clear, and again, she felt compelled to listen, even though the consequences this time were much steeper. Forcing her mind to overcome her heart, she broke off with Jordan and said good-bye to her dreams of the African wilderness. Brooklyn wasn't quite as exotic as Africa, but it was its own sort of jungle, one she's been navigating ever since.

∽ Chapter Nine ∽

Thursday was a busier day than usual. Dr. Robin, one of my colleagues, had recently moved to Boston after fifteen years at Bellevue. My schedule today was filled with Dr. Robin's patients, each of whom had mixed emotions about being assigned to a new doctor. No matter how brightly I presented myself, I could not be the six-foot-three dark-eyed physician with the soft-spoken midwestern charm and the meticulous pin-striped suits that they'd grown attached to over the years.

I reviewed the next chart, dreading the patient's impending disappointment that I had no way of avoiding. My heart sank even more when I noted the words *paraplegic* and *wheelchair*. Most of the patients I'd dealt with in this category were young men paralyzed from gunshot wounds related to gang violence and drugs. These were angry, difficult patients. Their issues of poverty, drug addiction, and sociopathic personalities remained with them, often festering in the aftermath of their injuries. If they weren't still using heroin or cocaine, many were addicted to pain medications. Distrust between patient and physician hovered like a low-hanging fog.

Jade Collier rolled herself to my office door with a sunny smile and a chipper "Hello" in that perpetually upbeat New Zealand accent.

I pulled away the chairs that my patients normally sat in, and she adroitly backed her wheelchair into the narrow space that remained. "You must be the new Dr. Robin," she said with the mock-serious style favored by late-night comedians. "'Tis amazing how he can make himself over."

Jade Collier looked younger than her fifty-five years, with short blond hair pushed casually behind her ears and impressively developed upper-body musculature. Most patients of her age that I'd seen in the clinic used motorized wheelchairs.

"Those people have given up, aye," she said with a sidelong glance. Her skin was freckled and tanned, lending her an outdoorsy air. "For me it's the use-it-or-lose-it philosophy."

I admitted that I'd never really thought about the manual-versus-electric-wheelchair issue.

"Oh, it's a huge debate in the community," Jade said, clicking the locks on her wheels. "There are those who believe you have to 'conserve it to preserve it,' but I think that's pure rubbish. They're just lazy." She tugged leather biking gloves from her hands and tucked them into the bag that was looped over the back of the chair. "I've never used a motorized chair, and I'll resist to the end," she said, and I could tell that she meant it.

I went through her medical history with her. Other than her injury, she was remarkably healthy: she didn't take any medicines, had no chronic illnesses. All of her rehab issues had been worked out years ago. She had enough upper-body strength to transfer herself in and out of the wheelchair independently. She could manage all of her self-care without assistance. She lived with her sister Katy, had helped raise Katy's children. These children now had babies, and Jade relished being a "grandmother."

As Jade told me how she was injured, I marveled at her composure. She told the story without any sense of anger, regret, or even sorrow. At first I attributed this to the decades she'd had to assimilate these facts of life—facts that were new and disturbing to me. But the more we talked, the more I saw that it was not simply an issue of the passage of time, it was more the nature of her personality.

I'd assumed that anyone with a devastating injury—particularly one that occurred so early, with such randomness, with such permanence—would possess a reservoir of anger or resentment, even if dulled over the years. But Jade did not appear to. Most of the recollections surrounding her injury, especially of her rehab, were surprisingly positive. Even accounting for the natural bias to recall positive experiences over negative ones, there was a genuine solidness to Jade that did not seem a façade.

"Do you ever dwell on the injury and those difficult years of recovery?" I asked.

"Oh, now and again I think about it," she said, leaning back in her chair. The leather exhaled a minor squeak. "There are occasional times where I cry and grieve, but it's not cathartic like you might expect." She paused for a moment, her eyes briefly distant. "It just is."

Over the years Jade had become very active in her church, and this was one of the main focuses of her life. This, along with her activism in the disability community, seemed to be bedrocks in her life.

"Sometimes these overlap," Jade said cheerily as we were finishing up the visit. "Just last month I converted my Access-A-Ride driver to Christianity." She gathered her things and unclicked the locks on her wheels. "You just never know when an opportunity for the Lord's work will arise!"

Jade maneuvered the wheelchair out of my office into the hallway as she bade me good-bye. I waved to her as she pivoted her chair to exit the clinic, surprised at how upbeat I was feeling, despite the busy day.

Although Dr. Robin's patients had been randomly assigned, I wanted to think of Jade Collier as a parting gift from him—not just because she spoke perfect English and was not weighed down by chronic illnesses, but because of the buoyancy that seemed to radiate from her. I called the next patient in, wondering if she'd notice the fresh, crisp air in my office.

∞ Chapter Ten ∞

One month later, I was back on the inpatient wards. The United Nations was having some sort of flamboyant celebration. I didn't know what the occasion was, and Bellevue Hospital was not an official part of it, but because we were only a few blocks down the road from the UN, we were the recipients of the fallout.

The scene in the hospital was not too dissimilar from what I imagined the General Assembly of the United Nations to look like. Envoys from the different nations were clumped in various locations throughout the ER, identifiable by distinctive dress and accents. There was the Ghanaian diplomat with acute gastroenteritis—his corner was the most colorful. There was the Pakistani attaché with an acute myocardial infarction—his cohort was huddled by the cardiac monitors in the ICU section of the ER. A Swiss nongovernmental worker had tripped off the curb—his group wore sleek double-breasted suits and spoke in whispers. The Estonians were louder, anxious that their undersecretary's migraine receive minute-to-minute monitoring. A Malaysian driver with an asthma attack sat in the "asthma corner," fifteen of his compatriots hunched over his nebulizer, fingering the tubing, inspecting the oxygen monitor.

When our team was up, we were assigned a twenty-six-year-old Tibetan hunger striker who'd been brought in against his will. Dawa Tenzin, we would learn later, had recently immigrated to the United States. He didn't speak a stitch of English, but he'd quickly been absorbed by the Tibetan émigré community. The Tibetans were out in full force during the UN celebration, protesting China's refusal to recognize Tibet and the ironfisted approach to the Tibetan democracy movement.

Mr. Tenzin had been on a hunger strike for almost a week, along with a group of monks and some fellow political activists. During a shouting match with some Chinese during a crowded human rights rally, Mr. Tenzin felt woozy and searched for a place to sit. Groping for a bench outside the mass of bodies, he became separated from his group, eventually staggering to the corner of East Forty-second Street. There, a policeman tried to assist him. Frightened by the touch of anyone in uniform, Mr. Tenzin bolted, but he only managed a few yards before he collapsed, and then an ambulance was called.

Now he lay on a gurney in the Bellevue ER, a rail-thin man with a shock of coarse black hair that spilled over his forehead. He looked wan from his hunger strike, but his eyes were vivid, frightened. Mr. Tenzin had ripped out the IV placed by the EMTs, and a bloodied bandage was all that remained on his arm. His two hands gripped the safety bars of the gurney, his knuckles pale from the compressive force. He looked as though he'd vault himself over the rails if he'd had the strength. There was no one in the ER who spoke Tibetan. Someone had called AT&T, but they didn't have an interpreter available at that moment. Call back in an hour, we were told.

Mr. Tenzin's blood pressure was low, 80/60, and his pulse was racing, indicating severe fluid depletion. His life wasn't in immediate danger but he needed urgent hydration and judicious refeeding. Within the first few hours of his fast, his body had run out of glucose and turned to the glycogen in his liver for energy. By the second day of his fast, the liver stores of glycogen had been depleted, and his body turned to the muscles for the glycogen it needed. Muscle glycogen lasted for another day or two, and then, to avoid cannibalizing the muscle protein, the body began to metabolize its fat stores, producing ketones—acetone-related compounds.

When we approached him with an IV kit, we could smell the fruity tinge of ketosis on his breath. As the intern began to sterilize his forearm for the IV, Mr. Tenzin pushed us away. I tried hand signals to indicate an IV in the vein and fluids flowing in, but he yelled something at me, a barrage of incomprehensible protest.

It was obvious that Mr. Tenzin didn't want our medical care. Because of the serious nature of his condition, it was imperative for us to assess his decisional capacity for refusal of treatment. More important, though, we wanted to convince him that he should stay in the hospital and accept treatment. I called back AT&T; still no interpreter available. Without an interpreter, Dawa Tenzin was isolated in an impenetrable bubble within the chaos of Bellevue.

An orderly with a crew cut and football-size biceps strode over and kicked loose the foot brake on Mr. Tenzin's gurney without a word. When the gurney began to move, Mr. Tenzin pulled himself upright, his eyes widening in panic, and began protesting again in Tibetan.

"Where are you going?" I demanded to the orderly.

"Seventeen Nawth," he snapped, his heavy Brooklyn accent completely eradicating the *r* of *north*. The tattoo on his left biceps said CANARSIE. "Bed's ready, and when the bed's ready we gotta get 'em up right away." He jerked his head toward the rest of the ER with its cacophony of international ills. "When the ER's backed up, they tell us to get our asses in action—pardon my French." He pushed Mr. Tenzin's gurney into the service elevator at a New York clip and our team scrambled along behind him.

The service elevator at Bellevue was a no-nonsense affair—industrial steel walls dulled from years of backs pressing up against them, a scuffed linoleum floor, harsh fluorescent lights, and a cranky Ukrainian elevator operator glued to a worn wooden stool. "Where to?" the operator grunted as we piled into the car.

"Seventeen," the orderly said. "Step on it."

The doors rumbled closed and the elevator lurched upward with a jolt. Mr. Tenzin was silent now, but his fear-stricken eyes darted jerkily from one corner of the elevator to the other. His fingers were still gripping the bars on the gurney, the muscles of his slender arms quivering from the effort.

The elevator operator sat hunched on his stool, head sunk into his shoulders, the collar of his jacket reaching the tops of his ears. He stared, unmoving, at the console of buttons directly in front of him. "They keeping you busy tonight."

I wasn't sure to whom he was talking, but the orderly answered. "ER's bustin' at the seams. This gotta be my twentieth trip, and my shift ain't half over." Now I could see the right biceps; it said DENISE.

The elevator operator continued to address the console in a monotone. "I hear that stuff's happening up at the UN, everybody knocking everybody over."

"Yeah, like this Chinese dude here," the orderly said, looking down at the patient on the gurney.

"He's not Chinese," I interrupted, annoyed. "He's Tibetan."

The orderly shrugged. "Chinese, Tibetan, whatevah. I just get 'em where they gotta go."

The elevator stopped to pick up an Indian phlebotomist laden with baskets of blood tubes. She was dropped off two floors later.

The elevator operator listlessly punched the buttons on his console to restart the elevator, never shifting his gaze toward any of us. "Tibet food's different from Chinese food," he said. "Less greasy, more soupy. That nurse aide over in pediatrics once brought me some Tibet food. She's a decent cook."

The elevator trundled to a halt on seventeen, and we all spilled out. The orderly hustled Mr. Tenzin over to his room, and I grabbed one of the medical students by the elbow. "Go down to pediatrics—it's on seven or eight, I can't remember which," I said. "See if you can dig up that nurse aide from Tibet."

Twenty minutes later, the student returned, jubilant at having located the sole representative of the Tibetan nation at Bellevue Hospital. The nurse aide was short—well under five feet—with a round face and silky black hair pulled into a tight bun. She was monumentally pregnant. The protuberant belly on her petite stature suggested dangerously unstable structural dynamics. Nevertheless, she moved nimbly.

Her last name was Dawa, Mr. Tenzin's first name. I walked beside her on the way to Mr. Tenzin's room, summarizing the issues that were of concern to us. She nodded but said nothing as I reminded her that we needed to assess decisional capacity, explicate the risks and benefits of refusing treatment, but also obtain informed consent for general medical treatment even if he was refusing specific treatments. Ms. Dawa nodded again and continued walking forward.

When we entered the room, the medical student quickly pulled up a chair for Ms. Dawa, as it didn't look like she could stay standing for much longer. When she dropped into the sagging chair, her head aligned right at the level of Mr. Tenzin's gurney.

She began speaking in a low, reedy voice, and the effect on Mr. Tenzin was immediate. His hands loosened their grip on the rails, easing themselves down onto the bed. The agitated corrugations on his face settled, and the terror in his eyes receded. His whole body seemed to sigh.

Ms. Dawa did most of the talking; Mr. Tenzin offered only occasional one-word answers. For fifteen minutes she spoke while the rest of us watched in silence. Ms. Dawa's voice resembled an oboe in the lower registers—air-filled, legato, haunting. It had a mesmerizing effect on all of us, including Mr. Tenzin, who slowly drew his hands together, letting them settle in a clasp over his chest.

Abruptly she stopped speaking, stood up, and turned to us. "You may proceed," she said. "There is no problem."

The nurse aide pivoted toward the door and we jumped to catch up with her. "What did he say?" I asked.

"He didn't say anything. I just told him about what I remember of Tibet when I was a little girl," she said as she walked back down the hall. "I reminded him about the beauty of our country and the mountains. I told him that the mountains would weep if we lost him." She pressed the button for the service elevator. "I told him that it was okay for the fast to be over. That it was okay to eat. That's all he needed to hear."

The doors opened—the Ukrainian elevator operator was still hunched on his stool, staring at the console. Ms. Dawa entered and leaned against the far wall, reaching one hand under her belly to support it. "He will be okay," she said, and then the doors closed.

When we returned to the room, Mr. Tenzin stretched his right arm out to us, resting his forearm on the metal rail. The intern pulled out a tourniquet and began prepping for an IV. Mr. Tenzin didn't flinch as the needle slid in. His eyes eased closed as the fluid entered his veins.

When I stopped by an hour later, one of the nurse aides was helping Mr. Tenzin with a bowl of broth. The aide was Jamaican, and she chatted amiably to her charge in patois, encouraging him to sip one spoonful after another. With each bite she cajoled—Mr. Tenzin hesitated, then accepted. And so it went, round after round, until the bowl was empty. The aide didn't let up her singsong Jamaican monologue for one moment. As I turned to leave, the aide raised an eyebrow at Mr. Tenzin, then tore open the top of the chocolate pudding with gusto. She rattled on, evidently with praises about Bellevue's pudding. Mr. Tenzin opened his mouth for a bite; it was clear that he understood.

It was well past dark when I walked home from the hospital that evening. The streetlamps of First Avenue created parallel orbs of light, illuminating the north–south artery. Looking uptown, I tried to convince myself that I could make out the United Nations, perched on a rise in the Manhattan topography just fourteen blocks from where I stood. The truth was that it was all a jumble of lights right now, but that didn't really matter. I knew that it was there, that microcosm of the world crammed into a monolithic office building. I often thought of the UN and Bellevue as sister organizations, both trying to cajole a Babel of cultures and languages into a comity of either the political or the corporeal sort. In any case, I was relieved that Mr. Tenzin was getting the medical care that he needed, that his body would finally be able to rest and perhaps his soul could too.

By the time I got home, supper was finished and the kids were already in bed. I tugged open the drawer in which we stowed the bounty of take-out menus that were edged under our door each day. I leafed through the menus for the local Afghani, Chinese, Thai, and Turkish restaurants. I put aside the Mexican, Japanese, Italian, and Moroccan ones. I knew there was a Tibetan restaurant in the neighborhood, sandwiched between a locksmith and the public library, but I hadn't eaten there. I sorted through the Indian, Pakistani, Vietnamese, and Peruvian menus until I finally found it. There were dumplings made of barley flour and yak butter, assorted stews, and curries. I settled on the savory soup with Himalayan daikon and bean-thread noodles. I ordered two portions, since I doubted that Mr. Tenzin's digestive system was ready for the eggs and dry toast that would likely show up on his breakfast tray tomorrow.

∽ Chapter Eleven ∽

Arzouma Érassa was a spry forty-one-year-old man with the slim build of a teenager. His face was smoothly spherical, glowing, and he had a thick, full Afro. He wore a seventies-style brightly printed yellow and purple shirt, reminding me of a young member of the Jackson Five. We spoke in French via the telephone interpreter, though he was able to respond to some of my questions in English before the interpreter translated them.

"Have you heard about what is going on in Togo?" he asked me on that Monday afternoon.

I was embarrassed to admit that I had not. I knew that Togo was a small country tucked somewhere in West Africa, but it didn't stand out in my mind. It hadn't been in the news, unlike Zimbabwe with its electoral violence and South Africa with its recent anti-immigrant murderous spree. Frankly, I couldn't recall ever reading or hearing anything about Togo. Was it one of those fiefdoms run by a maniacal dictator? Had it been economically decimated by colonial powers and left to wallow in poverty? Was it entrenched in endless civil war? Was it the battleground for proxy wars by distant superpowers? Or maybe it was one of those small, stable countries that somehow managed to hang on despite the generalized continental chaos? The last possibility was exceedingly unlikely, otherwise Mr. Érassa would not be sitting before me as a card-carrying member of the SOT program.

"I was interested in opposition politics ever since I was a student in our village," Mr. Érassa told me. "I wanted to stand up for freedom of expression, but I didn't want to fight. My friends called me a coward." He smiled as he said this, as though inwardly laughing gently at his younger self. "They made fun of me for being a weakling, but that was me—I just wanted to finish my studies, not run around in the jungle risking my life." When Mr. Érassa smiled, his cheeks rounded even more.

"It happened almost accidentally, ten years later when I went to law school. I was assigned an internship at the General Assembly.

This was my first introduction to members of the government." Mr. Érassa's face sobered. "I wasn't actually a member of the opposition party, but the government branded me as a member, and so that's how I started."

I nodded.

"They've always clamped down on anyone involved with the opposition," he continued, "arresting them and beating them." His hands underscored his words with restrained, precise gestures. "But a few years ago they started murdering them. They'd take them to a remote area at night, strap them in a car, then set the car on fire. The burned bodies would be found the next day."

His vivid eyes made appropriate contact with mine, but his voice contained a sadness that seemed distinct from depression—a profound sorrow and disappointment about his country. "They started sending out groups to 'interview' ordinary people. If the person said something they didn't like, they'd stab him on the spot. A friend of mine didn't know about this, and when he said he supported the opposition party they pulled out a knife and sliced open his abdomen. All the intestines came spilling out." Mr. Érassa didn't cringe or flinch when he told any of this to me. Even though this was clearly old news for him, there seemed to be an element of newly realized grief, as though he were still startled by the inventive brutality of the ruling party.

"My friend was lucky. He was smart and pushed all the intestines back inside. He held them there until he got to a Red Cross station, so he lived."

Mr. Érassa glanced away and I could see the fine muscles of his face tensing slightly, puckering the contours of his otherwise smooth visage. He paused for a long time, and I wondered if he was about to cry. I nudged my box of tissues out from under a stack of papers, but he ignored it. A finger and thumb reached up to the isthmus between his eyes, stanching any flow, real or imagined. The minutes ticked by, but Mr. Érassa seemed unaware.

Was it the image of his friend's intestines slithering out of his body that was fixed in his mind right now? I wondered. Was it something else? Or maybe it was no image at all—just a sense of bleakness. The background thrum of nurses, doctors, and patients passing by in the hallway trickled through the closed door as we waited out the silence.

"Two journalists were run down by cars at night," he finally said, voice tired, awkwardly patient. "The bodies were found in the morning, and it was said that it was an 'accident.' Other people were killed that way too. And I knew they would try to get me."

"Did they?" I asked.

"They ran me over with a car a week later," he said, looping his gaze back to me. His eyes were wide-set, prominent. "They left me for dead, but it only broke my legs. When I got better I applied for a visa to the United States, but everyone said that I would be arrested at the airport."

His main fear was for his wife, siblings, and elderly father, who might be harmed because of his political activity. "I hear they now just go right to people's homes at night and kill them. They don't even pretend to interview anymore." His wife had moved to a small village for safety, but that made phone contact all the more difficult.

I asked him how he was feeling now.

"Lonely," he replied, rubbing his palms over his knees. "In Togo, my wife and I had been trying to get pregnant, but we had trouble. We'd started seeing doctors, but now it may never happen because I don't know how long we will be apart."

I sat back and considered that. It was hard to imagine how people had time for ordinary worries, like bills, groceries, homework assignments, in a war zone, even an unofficial one. It seemed even harder to imagine being able to focus on infertility treatments—an issue that would seem to require a certain degree of personal, political, and economic stability. But the reality was that I was frankly ignorant—so much a product of societal happenstance that I hadn't the faintest conception of how one organized one's life and priorities in the face of psychosis on a national level. SOT was my weekly education.

"Sometimes I am forgetful and lose things," Mr. Érassa said with a hint of embarrassment in his voice. "My mind doesn't focus well. Sometimes I can't sleep and remember horrible things. It makes my heart race and my stomach hurt."

"Have you ever felt so sad that you would want to kill yourself?" I asked, as I was required to of anyone who offered symptoms of depression.

He shook his head with a pragmatic twitch. "No. I want to be
here for my wife. But if I were in Togo now, I might feel suicidal."

After Mr. Érassa, I saw that Samuel Nwanko was waiting for me.
He was again wearing sunglasses, hat, and denim jacket. When he
walked into my office, the anxiety of that first visit—my discomfort, his dashed expectations—flooded back. My hand clutched reflexively at the Styrofoam cup of water on my desk, but I resisted
the urge to pull it toward my mouth for a drink; I needed to clear
the air with him.

"Mr. Nwanko," I started, fingers gripping the cup, "I feel like
we—I—really disappointed you last time." I could feel the pliant
walls of the cup giving slightly from my grasp. "The things you
needed—specialized surgery, assistance for college—I couldn't help
you with any of them." My grip tightened and the cup threatened
to buckle. Yet I couldn't seem to let go.

When Mr. Nwanko dropped his head in a half nod, the brim
of his hat obscured most of his face. "I wish it were that simple,"
he replied, almost wistfully. "It would be easier to blame a person
or the system. But it doesn't solve anything. And you can call me
Samuel if you want."

His acknowledgment was as simple as it was generous.
Abashedly, I yanked my hand away before the cup crumpled completely and flooded my desk. I'd probably short-circuit the
computer and knock out the whole damn network.

"How are things going these days?" I asked, casting about for
a change of topic.

"I want to start applying for college," he said, "but everything
costs money. Even community college." Samuel looked up, and the
fluorescent lights glinted off his sunglasses, sparkling with an incon-
gruous festiveness. "The retreat where I'm staying is very generous
about me living there, but there's no money for tuition. I'm applying for jobs," he said. Then he hesitated. "But it's not going well."

I took a moment to contemplate the capacity of American society to set aside superficial appearances and consider the person beneath the face. I was not optimistic.

"How is your living situation at the retreat?" I asked, once again searching for a less fraught topic of conversation.

"It's fine, I guess." Samuel's hands sank together, palms facing inward, and slid into the gap between his knees as if seeking shelter. "The friars are very nice. They let me do my own thing. But last week, there was a—" He stopped midsentence.

I waited to see if he would continue. When he didn't, I asked, "Did something happen?"

He didn't answer right away, but his hands pressed deeper between his knees, canting his torso forward in an ever-narrowing angle until his gaze seemed to be riveted on a square of linoleum one foot in front of him. "Well, there are a few families who are also staying at the retreat. I don't sleep well—I haven't ever slept well since the attack—so I'm often up and about during the night." He slid even lower. "One night last week I wandered into the kitchen to get a snack. It was quite late. There was a boy there, from one of the families, and I guess he wasn't expecting anyone. Neither was I. But he got so scared . . . " Samuel's voice faded to a sibilant scratch. "So scared when he saw me that he screamed and then ran away."

The dryness crept back to my throat and my hand felt for the cup of water on my desk. I coaxed it slowly toward me, but when it was finally close enough to sneak an unobtrusive sip, it suddenly seemed rank and unappealing.

"I don't want to scare little children," he said. His voice was so soft I could barely hear it.

∽ Chapter Twelve ∽

Nazma Uddin was back on my list for the morning clinic session, weeks earlier than her scheduled appointment, but I was not surprised. She was always calling for extra appointments. The content of our visits rarely varied, but the frequency seemed to offer her some sort of comfort.

When I called her in from the waiting room, she came down the hall accompanied by a slender young woman cloaked entirely in black. A black head scarf covered her forehead, resting just above her eyebrows, and a thick black veil came up over the bridge of her nose, leaving the barest slit for her kohl-lined eyes—an even smaller space than in Mrs. Uddin's loose veil, which at least allowed her forehead to be exposed. The young woman's hands were encased in black linen gloves, and she moved like an apparition, with barely a rustle of her black robes. There was something both exotic and forbidding about her. I ushered the women in. As usual, Mrs. Uddin immediately unsnapped her veil, but the woman shrouded in black did not. I wondered if she was a relative visiting from Bangladesh.

"Good morning," I said. "How can I help you today?"

Mrs. Uddin's face was scrunched with frustration. She took out the bottle of antidepressants I'd prescribed at the last visit and plopped it on my desk. "These pills no good. They make veins in my neck swell. Fire burning in my head. No good."

"For how long did you take the pills?" I asked.

Mrs. Uddin waved away my question like she was swatting a fly. "I take few days, but no good. I need better pills."

If nothing else, Nazma Uddin offered consistency. Every visit was predictable. We tussled—gently—over the same issues, negotiated compromises that we'd tried before, and gave the whole thing another go. We'd been doing this for eight years now. I imagined us aging together, each offering the other a strand of stability.

"How are things at home?" I asked.

"Home good," Mrs. Uddin answered, the tautness in her face easing. She leaned toward the woman in black. "Azina visiting, so things good for this week."

Azina? This was Azina? Chubby, bespectacled Azina was now a slim high-school junior. At the mention of her name, Azina turned toward us.

"Mom," she said—and I could see her eyes roll within the tiny slit of her veil—"stop making such a big deal. It's just a visit, c'mon." Azina was attending a Muslim boarding school in upstate New York and was home for vacation. She slouched in the chair, and the cuffs of her jeans peeked out from under the edge of the gown.

"How is school?" I asked Azina, wondering about her transformation.

"Boring," she replied. "No boys in the classes, and they don't allow color," she informed me with perfect teenager ennui that immediately dissolved my initial forbidding impression of her.

I was intrigued by the differences between Azina's veil and her mother's. Mrs. Uddin's veil hung loosely over her face, like a curtain, and unsnapped with ease. Azina's was a black cloth pulled so tight that I could make out the contours of her nose, cheeks, and lips; it was tied somewhere in the back, under layers of her head scarf and gown. It looked vastly more uncomfortable to me, like it was smothering. She didn't remove her veil with me, and I wondered if that was because she had become more religious than her mother, perhaps as a result of her boarding-school experience.

As I contemplated this, it dawned on me how little I actually knew about the Muslim veil. No one in my personal life wore one. To be honest, the only information I had was from the news media and from seeing Muslim patients in the hospital; I had very little firsthand knowledge about Muslim dress. Perhaps it was time for me to learn.

I wasn't sure how sensitive a subject the veil was and wondered if it would be considered an affront to broach the issue. But I felt that I knew Mrs. Uddin—and, by extension, Azina—well enough by now, so I asked, somewhat timidly, if I might pose a question about the veil. They both nodded. I asked Azina if not removing her veil in my office like her mother did was a sign of increased religiosity.

Azina laughed uproariously as soon as the question left my

mouth. "No," she said, trying to control her ongoing snickers, "the only reason I don't take it off here is that it takes forever to retie and I'm too lazy. Just ask my mom!" Her ease with this, along with the magnitude of difference between my assumptions and her reality, relaxed the conversational berth. I felt comfortable now and asked all sorts of questions about the veil, even naïve ones. Azina took the lead in answering, her infectious energy spilling out despite the tight veil that completely wrapped her face. I wanted to know if it was hot under there. Was it hard to breathe? How did she decide what color, what style? Was it a family norm? Or did each mosque prescribe a different style? Did she wear it at home? What was the significance of the veils that draped low over the bridge of the nose and the ones that were tight up against the eyes? Did veil traditions in Bangladesh differ from those in other countries?

Azina and her mother chatted amiably, seeming delighted to educate me in the nuances of this aspect of Muslim culture. While the subject had been a little touchy for me, it certainly wasn't for them.

Taking a bit of a risk and pressing further, I asked if there was any pressure or coercion about wearing the veil. Mrs. Uddin answered this one emphatically. "No. Veil is my choice. My husband, he tell me not to wear it. He say people treat me bad, that they say I am terrorist." Her voice grew more animated and assured. "But veil is between me and Allah," she said, pointing upward. "I wear veil no matter what anyone say. It is my connection to Allah." The conversation proceeded toward Islam in general, and I learned how devout Mrs. Uddin was and what pleasure religious observance gave her.

The most interesting thing for me—besides all that I was learning—was the transformation that occurred in Mrs. Uddin. While discussing Islam and the veil, she became buoyant. All her whininess disappeared. The aches and pains seemed to evaporate. Her voice and body language reclaimed the heft and vitality one would expect from an otherwise healthy forty-three-year-old woman.

This was not a meek, oppressed woman, I thought. This was not a woman beaten down by a patriarchal religion. This was a woman inspired and fortified—dare I say empowered—by her religion.

I pointed out my observation of Mrs. Uddin's rapid improvement. Mrs. Uddin and her daughter were impressed, though not necessarily surprised. As I finished up my visit with Mrs. Uddin, I realized that we'd just gained a new clinical insight, and perhaps a new therapeutic tool. I realized that I might, finally, look forward to Mrs. Uddin's clinic visits. Although I didn't want her to keep Azina out of school for her appointments, I hoped that Azina would come to some of the visits so we could continue my education as well as her mother's "treatment."

My morning session always overlapped into the afternoon session, no matter how hard I tried to discipline myself to stay within the fifteen-minute slot for each patient. Sometimes it was due to fascinating conversations—as with Nazma Uddin and Azina—but mostly it was because of the ungainly sprawl of multiple chronic illnesses that the majority of my patients had. Thursdays were the busiest days of the week. I had patients all morning and then my weekly precepting session in the afternoon.

The fun part about precepting was supervising house staff with their patients. Each time a resident saw a patient, he or she would present the case to me and we'd discuss the diagnosis and treatment plan. Each case offered a small opportunity for teaching, but there were so many residents and their schedules were so complicated that we had only these—small moments. It was a stark contrast to the inpatient wards, in which we had a fixed team for a whole month with a dedicated ninety minutes of teaching rounds each day.

The not-so-fun part about precepting was everything else. The preceptor was the go-to person (some would say dumping ground) for refilling prescriptions, filling out forms, fixing scheduling snafus, reordering tests and labs whose requisitions had expired, dealing with panic values from the lab, handling abnormal results from radiology, and reviewing medication orders from visiting-nurse services—a nonstop array of ongoing annoyances.

The afternoon precepting session was well under way when I finally closed the chart of my last patient of the morning and relocated myself and my accoutrements—prescription pad, stamper, pocket medication guidebook, handful of pens, box of strawberries for the residents, sandwich that I hadn't had time to eat—to the precepting room. There was already a pile waiting for me—a mammogram needed to be reordered, a patient was confused about his hydralazine and his hydrochlorothiazide, a Celebrex prescription required prior authorization from the insurance company, a disability form needed to be filled out, a reflux medication wasn't covered by a patient's plan.

Two residents had already seen their first patients and were waiting to present to me. Luckily, they were senior residents and we could breeze easily through their cases—an Armenian man recovering from gout, and a Nepalese woman with diabetes and hypothyroidism. The interns' cases were more protracted affairs. The medical students' cases could be epic in length.

The clerk was already back with more. "Med refill," she said, adding a paper to the top of my pile. "He's here for oxycodone. Says his pills were stolen. Needs a new prescription plus a letter for the pharmacy, otherwise they won't refill it."

Medication requests for other doctors' patients were an irritation. Medication requests for controlled substances were purgatory.

I flipped through Tadeusz Kaczmarek's chart on the computer, and it wasn't very auspicious. He'd first gone to the ER five months ago, requesting medications for chronic pain related to spinal surgery done at Kings County Hospital. The ER gave him a week's supply and booked him an appointment with one of our residents. When he came to that appointment, he was given a month's supply of meds from the resident, who referred him to the pain management clinic and the neurosurgery clinic. Mr. Kaczmarek missed both appointments.

A month later, Mr. Kaczmarek came for refills. A month later, he came again for refills. A month later again.

Finally, Mr. Kaczmarek got another appointment with the resident. The resident rescheduled with pain management and neurosurgery. He gave Mr. Kaczmarek one last refill and said that no further prescriptions would be given until he saw these specialists.

That was three days ago. Now Mr. Kaczmarek was back. Stolen pills. Needed a doctor's letter for the pharmacy.

I could feel the anger begin to simmer at the base of my gut.

Why couldn't this patient be requesting something innocuous, like atenolol, instead of oxycodone? Why did he have to come on a day that his doctor wasn't here? Why did he have to put me in the position of having to decide whether or not he was telling the truth? Was he a disorganized patient who missed appointments and lost prescriptions, or was he a drug seeker or a drug dealer hustling us for narcotics?

More than anything, I wanted to shove the paper to the bottom of the pile and deal with it later. These messes were always dumped in the laps of the doctors. When I had confronted our administration about this, I was told that renewing controlled substances was "at the discretion of the doctor." Great advice. Thanks.

I reordered the mammogram. I explained the difference between hydralazine and hydrochlorothiazide. I filled out the disability form. I hunted through the fine print of the drug formulary for a reflux medication that was covered, though it took another ten minutes to decipher the three-tiered co-pay plan. I precepted three more cases, letting the discussion of the relative cardiovascular benefits of lipid lowering versus blood-pressure lowering go on a little longer than usual.

When I could avoid it no more, I steeled myself for confrontation and strode out to the waiting room. "Mr. Kaczmarek," I called out.

A scrawny man with craggy, ductile features and several days' of beard growth stood up. His hair was a worn shade of brownish blond, the top part cut short and spiky, the rest reaching to his shoulders. Thin, ropy arms protruded from a sleeveless T-shirt that depicted a rock band I'd never heard of. His denim jacket was tied tightly around his narrow waist. I beckoned him over to a corner of the waiting room where we could speak with some degree of privacy.

"Mr. Kaczmarek," I said, clipping my syllables to sound as dispassionate as possible. "You just got a refill of oxycodone three days ago, and now you're telling me that it was stolen?"

"I live in shelter," he said, jamming his thumbs into the sleeves of his jacket that formed a lumpy denim belt. "They steal all the time." His accent was a blend of Brooklyn and Poland.

"Your doctor has made several appointments for you to see the pain management specialists," I said tightly, "but you've missed them all."

"Shelter moves us all the time," he said, sniffing twice. His right hand pulled up from his waist, rubbed the side of his nose, then dropped back into its nook. "I moved from Bronx to Brooklyn, back to Bronx. All my papers lost."

The steam was rising inside my throat. Why couldn't he have given me a lamer story so I could just brush aside his request? Why couldn't he have confabulated something completely ridiculous? But no, he had to go ahead and say things that were entirely plausible: Shelter residents *were* constantly transferred between facilities. Theft *was* rampant. How was I to know whether he was being truthful?

The simplest thing for me, the easiest way to make the problem disappear, would be to take his words at face value and hand him a prescription along with a letter to the pharmacy that vouched for his story. I'd be done with it.

But the possibility that he could be using me to score more hits or make a quick buck infuriated me. I'd been dragged over the coals more than once by the plausible-story scam. Once, as a second-year resident, I'd sat in the ER pumping morphine into a freckle-faced young Canadian while the nurses derisively rolled their eyes. But the patient's story had been plausible, so I'd erred on the side of helping the patient, despite my doubts. Of course the nurses turned out to be right—the patient had been lying—and I was left with a hangover of embarrassment and anger.

But that's how they got you, with that plausible story. They milked you for the constitutional weakness that was built right into the Hippocratic oath—it was your *job* to help patients in pain, and they knew that. A doctor could be exploited on the very basis of his or her ethical commitment to patients.

I narrowed my eyes and gave Mr. Kaczmarek the once-over. He sniffed and rubbed his nose again. I dropped my gaze and scanned his forearms for track marks, but the light in this corner was too poor for me to tell. His hand went up a third time to rub his nose.

It was time to lay down the law, I decided. There were enough holes in his story to send this sociopath out the door. It was time to state unequivocally—at the discretion of this doctor, on behalf of all the doctors at Bellevue—that we would no longer give any narcotics to Tadeusz Kaczmarek. Then I'd pivot on my heel and retreat to the precepting room to document the official medical clinic policy according to Danielle Ofri, MD, in Mr. Kaczmarek's chart.

What if he really had been robbed? What if he really did miss his appointments because his life had been rendered completely ungovernable by the combination of poverty, homelessness, and illness, not to mention displacement from his native country?

Mr. Kaczmarek rubbed his nose again, and I was annoyed at the whole situation. "Did you report the theft to the police?" I asked, listening in disgust to myself sounding like a gumshoe in a B movie.

Mr. Kaczmarek pulled both arms out of his jacket and crossed them against his chest. "You no believe me?" he said. "You won't give prescription without police report?" He shifted his weight from side to side with mongoose-like tension.

"Well, if you were robbed you should have reported it," I said. I had started to sound defensive and I hated that.

"So, if I bring police report you give me prescription?" he said, taking a half step back, resetting the pulleys of his narrow shoulders.

Goddamn punk. Now I was backed into a corner. A police report wouldn't be proof that his medications were truly stolen; he could just as easily have lied to the police. But at least that would be evidence that he hadn't spun the whole story in twenty seconds in the waiting room. How far was I expected to go in this investigation anyway?

I gave a curt nod and stormed back to the precepting room. The whole thing made me feel nihilistic. If he was a drug dealer and I turned him down, he'd just go to another hospital, so I might as well have given it to him and saved myself this aggravation. But the idea that I might be a pawn in a drug scheme irritated me to distraction.

There was already a new pile of issues to address when I got back to my desk. Anatomic pathology needed a requisition for a urine cytology sample. A patient wanted a letter to get out of jury

duty. Vascular lab had called because a patient's Doppler was positive for a venous thrombosis. A visiting-nurse service needed authorization to get a walker for a patient. Three pharmacies had
left messages for prescription refills. A patient was ninety minutes
late for his appointment and the intern was refusing to see him. A
home attendant needed a letter saying she was medically cleared
to start work. A patient wanted a letter requesting a ground-floor
apartment because he couldn't climb three flights of stairs. Another
Viagra prescription needed prior authorization.

I fumed through the pile—stamping, signing, dialing—stopping
each time a resident came to present a case. I just hoped that none
of the house staff chose today to ask for career advice. I'd probably
have steered him or her toward accounting.

The next morning was a regular patient-care session. I wasn't the
preceptor for the clinic that day, but when I went out to the waiting room to call my second patient, there was Tadeusz Kaczmarek.
He spied me from his seat and hustled over, grasping a paper in his
left hand.

"I have police report, Doctor," he said, planting his toothpick
legs in their too-tight jeans in front of me. "You believe me now."
His right hand flew ever so briefly to his nose, and then shifted back
to his hair, pushing a few strands off his shoulder. His left hand
remained aloft with the police report. I snatched the paper and
unfolded it with a taut snap. It was a theft report from the Eighty-
third Precinct—signed, stamped, dated.

I glared at Tadeusz Kaczmarek—scraggly hair, shifty posture,
nervous tics. Of course he was trick-or-treating from hospital to
hospital getting oxycodone. Of course he was selling it on the
street. Of course he was an addict.

Except...except what if he wasn't? What if I was falling prey
to a stereotype? Even obnoxious, scruffy, homeless immigrants got
their share of diseases and legitimate pain.

The whole situation felt unseemly—the judging, the suspicions,
the hints of dirty dealings, the awkward power dynamics. I longed

for a clarity of crime, a simplicity of hate—but I was stuck with muck, and all I wanted was for this to be done with.

I pushed the police report back at him and leaned on the clerk's desk to write out the prescription. I avoided eye contact as I slid the oxycodone prescription and the letter for the pharmacy toward him. Swallowing back the sour taste in my mouth I slunk back to my office to start on my next patient.

Two minutes later a rapid-response code was called over the loudspeaker, and my body instinctively perked up. Somebody was having a seizure or difficulty breathing or plummeting blood pressure. Thank God. I bolted in the direction of the code, overjoyed to have something actually medical to deal with.

∞ Chapter Thirteen ∞

Every time I had a visit with a patient like Julia Barquero, with her complicated family history, or Señora Estrella, with her organic juicer, I reexperienced the frustrations of my limitations in Spanish. Though I did not possess a milliliter of Latino or Sephardic blood in my veins, my years at Bellevue Hospital had made Spanish a de facto second language and culture in my life. I observed bilingual staff members with palpable envy, jealous of their linguistic facility. I appreciated the "luck" of their circumstances (usually immigrant parents who kept Spanish alive at home while the children learned English at school). I regretted that my one opportunity for effortless bilingualism had been lost when my Israeli father found it too difficult to speak Hebrew to his fully Americanized children. I knew that I could never speak Spanish fluently until I lived in a Spanish-speaking country.

Over the years I'd privately been hatching a plan. We'd unmoor ourselves from our frenetic New York City lives and move to Spain or Mexico or Argentina for a year. I'd take a break from medicine and work on the novel that I'd always wanted to write. My husband would put aside software development and pursue his talent for art. We'd all immerse ourselves in a new language and culture.

But this dream seemed nearly impossible to fulfill. It wasn't just the usual excuses of complicated lives and difficulty uprooting. It was that Benjy and I were bound to jobs that had diametrically opposite rhythms. My working life was dictated by the rigid academic medical calendar, for which complex schedules of teaching, patient care, clinic supervision, ward supervision, and on-call coverage were arranged in fixed twelve-month blocks. Any time off would require nearly a year's advance notice. Benjy, by contrast, was an independent consultant. A project could finish—with little warning—on a Tuesday, and then he'd be available on Wednesday. He had no way to plan in advance, and I had no way to be spontaneous.

Nevertheless, I continued to nurture this fantasy. Maybe Ecuador. Maybe Bolivia. I'd heard that Santiago was beautiful.

What about Peru? But the motor that thrummed under my dream was that I wanted my children to have a chance at bilingualism. Naava was four and Noah two. At these tender ages, they could achieve, without so much as breaking a sweat, what I had been struggling with for years. It was a complete freebie for them. But it wouldn't be so later in life; I had to give them the opportunity when they where young.

So it was an odd planetary alignment of events that had us stroll into an open house on East Twenty-third Street one Sunday afternoon in November. We weren't looking to move from our rental apartment, but real estate window-shopping is a peculiar Manhattan obsession. The quirky layout of this loft, the period details of the former warehouse, and the uneven tin ceilings combined into a strange alchemy, and I was smitten. On a lark, we placed a bid. Luckily, some other soul had the good sense to outbid us by an extravagant sum and get us off the hook. But then the gears started to turn: if we had considered extracting our life savings for an apartment (nothing more than four walls, really), what else might we use that money for? Why not for that coveted year abroad?

The start of the medical academic year was still eight months away, possibly enough time to apply for a leave of absence. Benjy's current project was beginning to reach its closure. What if he took on only short-term projects for the next few months?

I attacked the many levels of bureaucracy in my hospital. I cashed in my seventeen years' worth of chits—seven years as a student, three as a resident, seven more as a faculty member. The administrators had mixed feelings about my request but were by and large supportive. I worked with them to find a temporary replacement in the clinic. I spoke to most of my patients and drafted letters in English and Spanish for any others who might turn up later and be surprised by my absence. I submitted documentation in triplicate and quadruplicate. I obtained signatures and approvals from all and sundry. I placed holds on my computer passwords and voice mail and hospital e-mail. We renegotiated our contract at day care and made arrangements for our apartment. I researched international animal transport requirements—we of course had to include our dog, Juliet, in this adventure. We obtained passports for Naava and Noah. In the end, I received permission from the hospital for a one-year unpaid leave of absence. I was ecstatic.

The exciting part was exploring different countries, different settings, options for the children. Would we go to Central America, South America, or Spain? We tried on different fantasies of living in a remote rain forest, on an undiscovered beach, on a cliff overlooking a canyon, in a small mountain village tucked away from civilization. We'd be newcomers in a new world. We'd plunge into the full experience, not as tourists but as real people living real lives. We'd knit ourselves into the local culture. Our children would attend the local school. We'd shop in the markets, adopt the cuisine. We'd spend a year far from American television, fast-food chains, crass commercialism. We'd leave the old world behind and integrate ourselves into a new one. We'd bind ourselves to the simple life.

And then I discovered I was pregnant.

The first thing my mother-in-law said, sensibly, was "You're going to cancel your trip, right?" Our first two children had been born in my hospital, two blocks from our apartment. There was security in the familiar—familiar hospital, familiar doctors, familiar health-care system, our own home, not to mention the convenience of being able to sprint the hundred yards to medical help if needed. But by now we'd invested so much effort—both logistical and emotional—into carrying out this plan of living abroad. I didn't want to shortchange our new child, but I also couldn't bear to part with this dream, knowing that life grows ever more complex and that this opportunity might not arise again. There had to be a way to continue with this while also ensuring safe circumstances for the baby.

We decided to soldier on. The prospect of delivering a baby in another country streamlined our thinking. Now we wouldn't live in the unblemished remote jungles, and we'd have to take the health-care system into account when selecting a country. Costa Rica turned out to be the best choice. We found a place to live that was removed enough from the city for us to enjoy the natural beauty, but still close enough for us to get to a reputable hospital.

We arrived in Escazú, Costa Rica, that July—me, four months pregnant, with a four-and-a-half-year-old daughter, a two-and-a-half-year-old son, a seventy-five-pound black Lab mutt, eight duffel bags, two laptops, and a cache of bug spray. I thought about how my patients arrived in their new homeland—Julia Barquero crossing a desert on foot from Guatemala after leaving her baby behind; Samuel Nwanko, sightless, on a plane from Nigeria accompanied by the young girl with a cleft palate who spoke no English; Aristide Mezondes arriving from Congo by boat with only his rudimentary Spanish to help him navigate America.

I thought about my maternal grandfather sailing across the Atlantic as a teenager with only his brother, navigating Ellis Island, setting up a fabric cart on the Lower East Side. They had all journeyed and had all arrived—under circumstances that I couldn't even begin to contemplate. I was getting to do it the easier way.

Because of flight delays, we had arrived in our new home in the darkness of the night. There was nothing to do but go to sleep. Several hours later, I was awoken by a chorus of staccato birdsongs. It was as though a woodpecker initiated a bass-line rhythm, but then the song was taken over with a distinctive lilting arpeggio. I opened the window and gazed into the dawn of our first Costa Rican morning. In front of our house was a knot of statuesque ficus and cedars, interspersed with willowy palms and trees sporting leaves the size of dinner plates. Brilliant flowering bushes offered a full palette of reds, yellows, greens, and oranges. Dense, snaking vines filled in all available space between trees, bushes, houses, and roofs.

The edges of everything before me were blurred by dew, and there was a layer of fog that carpeted the valley below. A lush verdant aroma filtered in through the window, then the silence was again punctuated by the staccato arpeggio song. A swish of movement identified the chanteur—a compact black bird whose tail fanned out during flight to reveal a dramatic golden underside. First one, then another, then a third swooped across the sky, a canon of flight and song. These were the aptly named oropendola, and they became our daily alarm clocks.

I was eager to meet our Tico (Costa Rican) neighbors, eager to learn about the new society we had planted ourselves in. I figured that I'd have a few weeks to settle in, explore the health-care system, check out the local hospital, figure out who would be the right obstetrician for me. But, as with many things in life, children do not permit the luxury of leisurely pacing.

Costa Rica offers an abundance of tropical fruits, and we were excited to try the many unusual varieties—*mamón chino, granadilla, jojote, guayaba, maracuya, cos, cherimoya.* On our fourth day in the country, my son, Noah, discovered that the smooth seed of the *guanábana* fruit fits perfectly up the nostril of a little boy. Benjy was out with our rental car trying to buy a refrigerator, we had no cell phone, and I was home alone with my two young children. I could touch the bulge of the seed near the bridge of his nose, but I couldn't figure out a way to extract it.

I did a mental survey of my situation, debating if it was time to panic: there was a foreign body in my son's nose that could easily be aspirated into his lungs. We were newly arrived in a foreign country. I didn't know my neighbors. I didn't have a cell phone connection to my husband. I didn't have a car. There wasn't a hospital two blocks away—in fact, I had no knowledge of what lay two blocks away. I didn't yet know the phone number or location of the hospital I'd planned to have my baby. I didn't know if there was a 911 system in Costa Rica. While I spoke passable Spanish, I wasn't sure of my ability to explain a *guanábana* seed up the nose. Yes, I was a doctor, but without medical supplies, nursing staff, medications, resuscitation equipment—being a doctor in an isolated situation wasn't going to be useful if the seed traveled to his lungs.

I did the only thing I could think of—I phoned home. If there was one phone number that was irrevocably seared into the gyri of any doctor who'd ever trained at Bellevue, it was x3015—the ER. I picked up my phone in Costa Rica and dialed the Bellevue Hospital emergency room.

"Hi, this is Dr. Ofri," I said casually, as if I'd just been paged from the Sixteen North medical ward. "I'm calling from Costa

Rica. We're experiencing a minor tropical emergency—there's a *guanábana* seed in my son's nose and I can't get it out."

There was silence on the other end of the line, and then a hesitant voice. "I'm sorry, could you repeat that again?"

Those ER clerks were supposed to be unfazable. Meanwhile, I was pressing my brain to recall the child-and-infant CPR course that I'd taken years back. For aspiration did you flip the child over onto your thigh to do back blows, or was it chest thrusts from the front? Did you do CPR with one hand or two?

I was eventually transferred to the pediatrics side of the ER. I explained the story again to another clerk. I was put on hold again and was now starting to lose patience. Yes, the story sounded sort of goofy, but what if Noah did aspirate the seed? What if my two-year-old son suffered a respiratory arrest in a foreign country that I'd dragged my family to because of some sort of fantasy of learning Spanish?

Finally I was connected to a pediatrics intern who was probably seventy-two hours out of medical school. The intern put me on hold yet again while he presented the case to his attending. The way to dislodge a seed from the nose, he instructed me when he returned, was to press the other nostril closed and blow out as hard as you could. But if you couldn't explain how to do that to a toddler, you had to blow it out for them, essentially performing mouth-to-mouth resuscitation.

I laid Noah on the floor, with Naava and Juliet crowding in to see what was happening. I occluded Noah's unaffected nostril, placed my lips over his, and blew as hard as I could. Needless to say, both Naava and Noah found this hilarious, giggling uncontrollably, making it difficult for me to maintain the tight seal I recalled from CPR training. Juliet began howling, licking, and nosing her way into the action, while I tried to remain composed. The *guanábana* seed turned out to be a tenacious little thing, not amenable to coaxing massage or mouth-to-mouth resuscitation. Luckily, Noah's respiratory status remained stable. Benjy returned home—sans refrigerator—and we obtained directions to the local hospital after knocking on a neighbor's door.

This last part—directions—may sound like a small thing, but

in Costa Rica it was anything but. For all its advances in so many aspects of society, Costa Rica was surprisingly quaint when it came to roadways. The combination of cheap pavement materials along with the annual rainy season that flooded the roads for weeks on end served to pucker and pockmark roads with potholes larger than many Manhattan apartments. The streets were windy and perilously narrow, lacking any sort of shoulder (ditches and cliffs were more common), and filled to bursting with two-way traffic of buses, trucks, bicycle riders, and cows. But the abysmal quality of the roads was only the beginning of the driving challenge in Costa Rica.

There were no street signs to be found; not a single road was labeled. But of course, there weren't any street *names* either, so lack of signage was superfluous. No one could offer me an explanation for this—it was simply the way it was.

As a result, direction-giving was a complex art form that typically involved such open-ended expository suggestions as driving five hundred meters to the mango tree, turning right where the post office used to be, circling around the pothole near the house with the blue fence, and so on.

It wasn't just that those of us from the nontropical climes might not be able to distinguish a mango tree from a *guayaba* tree from a *jojote* tree; or might not know where the former post office had existed or that the blue fence had been painted green in 1973; or might not be aware that five hundred meters was a Rorschach-like estimation of distance that bore only a fleeting resemblance to that of the European Union Metric Standards. It was that fully half of the proffered directions were simply incorrect. Everybody was eager to provide directions. Whether people actually knew where the destination was had no bearing on their willingness to offer intricate and idiomatic directions. In our entire year, I never met a single person who said "I don't know."

Armed with a dissertation's worth of directions, we piled the family into the rental car and ventured forth, me with one hand on Noah's wrist to monitor his pulse. We bumbled our way past the landmarks of the *fruitería* and what we hoped was a mango tree and onto the directionless highway. The exit for the major hospital—like the one leading to the international airport—was pristinely unblemished by signs. Luckily, the roadside flower stand—the landmark for our exit—was open and doing a brisk business on that warm July day.

Since this was the hospital in which I intended to give birth, I was happy to see that it was clean and modern looking. The registration, however, seemed endless as I painstakingly filled out the forms in Spanish. Many sections stumped me, such as address. Given the country's casual attitudes toward street names, it should have come as no surprise that addresses in Costa Rica were not paragons of exactitude and that mail delivery offered the same suspense as the scratch-off lottery games. When we'd signed the rental agreement for our house, the address was listed as *300 metros al sur del Supermercado La Flor, Casa #2.* Was that what I was supposed to write on this hospital registration form—that we lived in the second house three hundred meters south of the dingy corner store that passed for a supermarket?

The registering clerk pointed out a section on the form that required my *número.* I pulled out my health insurance card from my wallet, but she waved it away. I offered my Social Security number, but she shook her head. She said what sounded like *citizen's number.* I explained that we weren't citizens, that we were visitors but that we were living here, at least for the moment. Meanwhile I was getting anxious that these forms were taking so long and my son still had a *guanábana* seed crammed up his nose. Who knew what sort of toxins were leaching out into his mucous membranes while we were debating about citizen numbers and *supermercados*? Who knew how soon the seed was going to travel to his lungs while I was failing test after test in this clerk's eyes?

Finally she asked for my passport number. My passport, of course, was at home, where it was supposed to be, safely tucked away with our plane tickets, and I didn't know the passport number by heart. The clerk shot me an exasperated look. By that point I just wanted to grab Noah's hand and march right in. I knew my way around emergency rooms; I knew the language of medicine and the hierarchy of hospitals. I was on my home turf here—I could break right in and get this situation solved.

But I wasn't on my home turf. There was nothing I could do but bottle up my complicated feelings of inadequacy, frustration, anxiety, and impatience, and wait for our forms to be processed. We sat in the waiting room with all the other patients and families. The news burbled on in Spanish on an overhead TV, captivating the entire room but us. I kept my eyes trained on Noah, watching for any change in respiratory status. At least we were *in* a hospital, should anything happen.

Finally a nurse called us in. Her rituals of blood pressure and temperature were familiar. We waited in a cubicle until the ER doctor arrived. She gamely spoke to Noah in the little English that she knew, but that comfort soon became irrelevant. When she pushed the long-nosed hemostat clamp up Noah's nose to extract the seed, Noah's screams dominated everything. I squeezed twenty pounds of squirming boy in my arms, trying to hold him still to allow the metal tool higher and higher still. After five excruciating attempts, defeat was admitted.

We were referred to an ENT specialist in the adjacent building whose office hours, thankfully, hadn't yet ended. We trooped over to his waiting room and settled into a new set of chairs. When I glanced up at his door, something caught my eye—a mezuzah. A strange feeling of comfort came over me. I didn't know this doctor and surely didn't think he was more qualified because he was Jewish. But it was something familiar in a strange place, and I felt a few degrees less lost.

Dr. Guzman-Marrero was a genial physician of Bolivian descent. His English was fluent though formal, and he quickly settled Noah into a comfortable exam chair. While he laid out an array of surgical tools on the metal stand, I kept reminding Noah about the promised ice cream that would surely materialize after this procedure. I hoped Dr. Guzman knew of the nearest vending machine.

"There will be no need for machines—vending or otherwise," Dr. Guzman said, spraying a quick dose of anesthetic inside Noah's nose. "You will find the hospital restaurant rather sufficient. I have full faith that ice cream exists on the menu."

He had Noah's attention by this point. "There is vanilla, no doubt," the doctor continued. A small retractor widened Noah's nostril. "Chocolate, I can offer personal guarantees." He positioned the light. "Strawberry is a distinct possibility." He adjusted the mirror. "Often there will be mango or guava." A narrow forceps wended its way up. "But for sure"—Noah winced and squeezed his eyes tight—"there are ice cream cones." The *guanábana* seed slid out onto a waiting gauze pad like a prize from a bubble-gum machine.

Dr. Guzman wiped the seed dry and handed it to Noah, who eyed it warily, then snatched it and crammed it into his pocket. We thanked the doctor profusely and followed his directions to the hospital restaurant. His predictions were all true, and now we all knew two words in Spanish—*guanábana* and *helado*.

Thanks to friendly neighbors, we were able to settle into our small house, acquire basic furniture, locate the weekly vegetable market, find a preschool for Naava and Noah, and learn when the fish man came around with fresh *corvina* in the trunk of his ancient Nissan. Through Peruvian friends we found a homey *ceviche* restaurant that came with an old swing set and a river in the courtyard. It quickly became a family favorite. We found local music teachers and began violin and cello lessons. We found the best parks for bike riding, and Naava and Noah became proud owners of their very first bicycles. We learned the ins and outs of the supermarkets—which ones gave free samples of cheese, which ones let you pay your phone bill there.

Our major purchase for the year was a car. As city dwellers, we'd never owned a car, and our lack of automobile savvy was glaringly apparent. Needing space for two kids, the dog, and an upcoming baby, we opted for a van. Not wanting to spend too much money on a one-year vehicle, we settled on one that might charitably be called "secondhand," bought from an outgoing missionary. The van was christened Juan Carlos the Sixty-seventh by Naava and Noah, to honor the sixty-six previous lives it had obviously had. We soon learned the phone number of the local mechanic. We quickly appreciated the importance of putting his phone number on speed dial. We soon learned the word for tow truck—*grúa*.

One day we visited the Poás volcano. We had been told to do any sightseeing early in the morning, before the afternoon rains started. Getting small children out the door, even for a day trip, is a major affair, and we left later than we should have.

The drive up hadn't been too bad, maneuvering Juan Carlos through the winding, potholed roads. The narrow roads lacked any sort of guardrails to protect against the precipitous drops, but the stunning mountain views kept our minds off the danger.

Set amid mountains laden with lush coffee plantations, Poás was a hauntingly stark, lunarlike crater, with strange outcroppings and jagged beauty. The winds whipped through the mountains, pressing in thick clouds then shooing them away with cinematic rapidity. As the day wore on, the clouds grew heavier and more dense, lower to the ground. It was time to leave.

For the first half hour of the return trip we drove directly through the cloud. With Juan Carlos's weak headlights, we could see nothing but the fog in front of us. As raindrops precipitated from the vapor, the cloud thinned. Soon it evaporated into pure rain. As we wended our way down the steep mountainside, the rain grew steadily heavier until it reached torrential proportions. When I'd first arrived in Costa Rica, I'd wondered at the lack of sidewalks, but now I understood why roadside ditches were far more practical. I watched the furious swells of water in the adjacent ditches with growing apprehension. There seemed an agitated force of nature—both mesmerizing and terrifying—restless in the human-built constraints. When the water finally surged over the craggy edges of the ditches and began sliding in vast sheets across the roadway, my anxiety started to crest.

The feeble wipers of Juan Carlos sloshed water across the windshield, clearing nothing. Visibility was no more than a few feet. Water and rocks pummeled the tires of the van, testing the treads and brakes that we had every reason to have little faith in. Mud gushed with the water as everything—including us—followed the relentless downhill course.

Questions began stalking me as the pace of the weather and the water picked up. What on earth had possessed us to undertake a trip on such treacherous roads in a car that counted duct tape as one of its key safety features? Why weren't we home in New York doing normal things with our children, like playing in playgrounds with padded mats or driving them in streets that had functioning storm drains? And if there was this much flooding at the top of the mountain, what exactly would be awaiting us when we reached the bottom?

Our fears getting the better of us, we made a sharp turn into a random driveway and parked in front of a house. We sat nervously in the car as shimmering sheets of rain surged down the mountainside, trying to decide if we were the overreacting tourists who panicked at the slightest native experience or the wise travelers who were sensible enough to detect danger and act accordingly. Torrents of rain battered the roof with a percussive force that made it difficult to hold a conversation. The cracked rubber door seals permitted a steady stream of water to seep inside the car.

I couldn't keep down the growing sense that things were beyond our control, that events of nature and the realities of this foreign country would determine the outcome of this day, not us. At that moment, I had a deep and overwhelming longing for the calm of New York City.

Another half hour went by. The rain showed no sign of letting up and we wondered if we'd be spending the night in the driveway of strangers. Benjy finally ventured out of the car into the deluge to knock on the door of the house. My husband has many talents, but, inconveniently, Spanish is not the best developed of them. Still, he made creative use of gestures and managed to get the questions across: Is this normal? Are we in danger? The gist of the family's reply was *It's the rainy season; this is rain!*

In retrospect we should have figured that a country known for its rain forests would be heavily endowed with rain, but as newcomers, we simply hadn't comprehended what rain could entail.

I thought about my patients and how they had braved circumstances far more challenging than this and with far fewer resources. I had a newfound respect for how frightening it must have been for them to arrive in a strange country and face unexpected obstacles. I craned my neck and glanced behind us. Naava and Noah were strapped into their car seats, chomping away obliviously on hunks of dried *piña* that mercifully never seemed to dissolve. Beyond them was a slow but steady stream of fifth-hand Citroëns and Toyotas—tiny four-cylinder cars—trundling their way up and down the flooded mountain road. Benjy and I looked at each other. If those beat-up wrecks could do it, certainly our beat-up wreck could. We threw Juan Carlos into reverse and backed out of the driveway. When in Rome, drown like the Romans.

∽ Chapter Fourteen ∽

The first thing our children grew to love in Costa Rica was the postage-stamp-size playground next to our house. There were two swings, one narrow slide, and a small wooden tower to climb on. From the upper reaches of the tower, both Naava and Noah could yank the green-skinned *limón dulce* from the overhanging tree. Despite the name, the fruit wasn't sweet, although it wasn't as sour as a regular lemon. But the Nicaraguan and Costa Rican babysitters plucked these for their hungry charges, and our kids followed suit. They grew accustomed to the flavor and soon got the hang of peeling off the thin, friable skin. Snack time was as simple as reaching up to the nearest tree.

In those first few weeks, Naava and Noah were adjusting to a preschool in which all the teachers spoke Spanish. At first they were miserable, and we were faced with the daily heart-wrenching decision of whether to press our crying children into the hands of the waiting teachers. The teachers encouraged us to be patient and promised us that we were not harming our children.

Before the end of the first month, we noticed that when Naava and Noah played together, they seemed to babble in gibberish, making up their own words that were neither English nor Spanish. But when I paid closer attention, I realized that their gibberish exhibited perfect Spanish intonation. They rolled their *r*'s, accented their *l*'s, widened their vowels, adapting the singsong pattern of Spanish even though they weren't saying any actual Spanish words.

It must have been in our second month one evening when Benjy was struggling with the fine print of the Spanish-English dictionary. "What's the word for rabbit?" he asked me. "*Vaca?*" Before I could answer, a squeaky voice piped up from the far corner of the room.

"*Conejo,*" said Noah, head still bent down toward the puzzle he was assembling, sippy cup gripped in his right hand. "Rabbit is *conejo,*" he repeated for emphasis. "*Vaca* is cow!"

It took a few moments to realize what had just taken place. But there was our son—roughly two months out of diapers—informing us how to properly identify farm animals in Spanish.

Naava's and Noah's acquisition of English had been intimately tied to their neurologic acquisition of language, so it had unfolded gradually over the course of two years. But with Spanish, it was like watching the fast-forwarded movie of an unfurling flower. Over mere weeks and months, we witnessed a new language take root in a completely natural manner. They had no difficulty with the concept of two words for every object around them. They didn't study vocabulary lists or conjugation tables like we did and they didn't go out of their way to practice Spanish like we did. But when they wanted to play with their German friends across the street, or when they wanted ice cream from the local store, or when they wanted to talk with their classmates at school, they knew that Spanish was the only way to do it, and so they spoke it, without any grammatical self-consciousness—and with an accent indistinguishable from any Tico's.

I pursued weekly Spanish lessons with Rigoberto, a local teacher around the corner from the *fruitería*. Rigoberto converted his living room into a classroom by installing long wooden desks with attached benches in the style of a one-room schoolhouse. At every lesson, Rigoberto wore a silk tie and a cardigan. On the first day, he covered the board with a list of twenty idiomatic phrases. "Americans sound American," Rigoberto said, "because they speak like a textbook."

Rigoberto was determined to purge my Spanish of its Spanglish. When I told him that at Bellevue we used the verb *chequear* when we wanted to check labs or check a blood pressure, his face drained of color.

"*Chequear* is not a word," he said, mouth tight with indignation.

"Even the native Spanish speakers in the hospital use it," I said.

"Barbarians," he spat. "Can't even speak their own language." He pushed a dictionary across the wooden desktop. "Go ahead. Look it up."

The Instituto Español dictionary was four inches thick. I paged through it, laboriously scanning page after page in the *ch* section. He was right; *chequear* wasn't there.

"*Re-vi-sar,*" he articulated, pounding a first with each syllable. "*Revisar* is the proper word. Don't listen to those philistines from the Caribbean."

Though I labored mightily over my Spanish lessons during the course of the year, I realized that a crucial element was missing for linguistic immersion: practicing medicine. If I weren't in a situation in which I was forced to speak Spanish every day, all day, with people who did not speak English, I would never achieve what Naava and Noah were achieving.

For the adults in our community—a mix of Dutch, Italian, German, Mexican, Russian, Australian, and Costa Rican—English was often the easier common language because most people used English in their work life. If they didn't, then they desired to improve their English because of its necessity. But for the children, Spanish was the only language available in order to successfully play tag, hide-and-seek, or blocks.

Toward the end of our year, we took a trip to Arenal volcano with my in-laws, who were visiting Costa Rica. We stayed in a tiny cabin, which lacked a phone. When my mother-in-law wanted to call home, Benjy took her to the owner's cabin where the sole phone was located; Noah tagged along. The owner did not speak English, and in the end, it was three-year-old Noah who became the fulcrum of communication, translating back and forth for his father, grandmother, and the hotel owner with enough accuracy to resolve the confusion.

My Spanish got a daily workout negotiating the quotidian essentials of living and traveling. But the thoughtful conversations and the friendships took place in English. It wasn't quite what I'd hoped for—linguistically at least—but still the year was a special and worthwhile experience on all fronts, even beyond the fact that we'd arrived with two kids and would get to return with three.

I was excited about starting cello lessons in Costa Rica with a local teacher. I learned about a vibrant music scene—seven orchestras in a country of four million, abundant concerts and festivals. "Costa Rica does not have an army," my teacher Sergio told me, "but it does have violins." Music lessons also seemed like an ideal and practical venue for improving my Spanish. But Sergio requested that we speak English so that he could use our lessons to work on his English along with my bowing and intonation. He had done part of his musical training in Germany, however, so German words frequently tumbled out inadvertently. One time when I was playing a Bach march rather lugubriously, he leaned over and said, *"Schnell, schnell!"* My bow froze on the D string as an involuntary shudder ran through me. He probably had no idea that a Jewish American who was well steeped in World War II documentaries would have such a visceral reaction to that word. He, of course, merely wanted me to play faster, at the indicated allegro tempo, and his brain translated more quickly into German than English.

The best part about cello lessons was that they took place on our veranda. In fact, most of our life that year took place on that veranda. Smooth red tile floor with a terra-cotta roof, the space had been built as a carport. Instead, it became our living room, and Juan Carlos was relegated to the cobblestone street.

Exuberant branches of magenta bougainvillea spilled over the edges of the roof, creating the feeling of a nest within which we arranged the simple wicker furniture. A cage of chirping parakeets, bequeathed to us by our Dutch neighbors down the block, hung under the flowering boughs and added an ongoing layer of song. Juliet spent her entire year splayed out on the sunny path to the veranda, retiring under the roof only when the afternoon rains began. For a New York City stray who'd spent her puppyhood in a pound and then the rest of her life in an apartment, it must have seemed as though she'd stumbled on nirvana. For the humans in the family, it had that sense as well.

In the sunny early mornings, we'd eat breakfast in the cool shade of the veranda. Rainy afternoons were almost more wonderful; in New York City, rain equaled "indoors," but here we could still play outside during the rain, creating elaborate play-dough projects on the veranda table while waterfalls gushed just a few feet from us.

On clear days, the central valley of Costa Rica stretched before us, encircled by a ring of mountains. We hung the requisite hammock, and when I wanted to fulfill Costa Rica's unofficial motto of *la Pura Vida*, I'd stretch out in that hammock with a bowl of sliced mango, listen to the fugue of the parakeets and oropendola, and watch the clouds shift lazily from purple to blue to deep azure as they wafted across the mountains.

It was at these moments that I was suddenly cognizant of the magnitude of stress woven into our New York City lives. While engaged in that life, I wasn't attuned to the sheer effort required to balance doctoring, parenting, and writing. Even as I relished all of these facets of my existence, I wasn't able to perceive the cost in energy and spirit. It was only when I had stepped away, relinquished medicine, that I could experience a beautifully bearable lightness of being. I was able to fit music and writing into my day, not cram it into late nights and weekends. I wasn't rushed with my children, or my meals, or my showers, or my conversations. There was time to socialize, to read, even to daydream.

I was fully conscious that this peaceful interlude had been made possible by giving up our jobs, by living off savings, that this was somewhat artificial and absolutely temporary. Nevertheless, it was a tranquil repose in our lives, and I didn't take one single moment of those 365 days for granted. What surprised me the most was that I did not miss medicine. Although I felt so strongly connected to my patients and believed that my colleagues were truly the cream of the crop, there was not one day of those 365 that I gazed out at the Costa Rican valley and wished I were going to Bellevue. I loved my job at Bellevue, had spent my entire professional career at Bellevue, yet it seemed so tantalizingly simple to let it all float away. Had a magic benefactor materialized and offered lifetime financial stability, I could have envisioned staying in Costa Rica forever, easily occupying my time with writing, music, and family. Part of me was horrified that medicine, this pillar of my life, could evaporate so blithely, but another part of me just wanted to wink at the bougainvillea, peel my papaya, and lie back in that hammock with one foot resting on Juliet's sun-warmed fur.

⸻᙭᙭᙭⸻

My pregnancy was progressing well. I'd found an obstetrician I was comfortable with—Dr. Agosín-Buksztajn, a soft-spoken Uruguayan Costa Rican. Thanks to fellowships in Boston and Haifa, he was fluent in English and Hebrew as well as Spanish. Though I tried to speak Spanish at our first visit, I found myself too embarrassed to be making grammatical errors in front of an educated person and soon abandoned my efforts.

I felt well cared for in Dr. Agosín's practice. Even more, I felt well cared for in the country of Costa Rica, which exuded a child-friendly attitude I'd never seen in America. The first time I entered a bank to change money, I pulled out a magazine to read while I waited on the snaking line. My reading was disrupted when I felt my arm being gently but urgently tugged. It was the guard from the front door. He pulled me out of the line, pointing to another window at the far end of the bank. Pasted on top was a sign with one schematic drawing of a parent with two children and another of an obviously pregnant woman. As he pulled me in that direction—he didn't even bother speaking, assuming that I must be a foreigner if I didn't know these rules—I came to understand that the bank offered a special window for pregnant women and parents with small children. Chairs were lined against the wall so we could sit while we waited. I was almost embarrassed to leave the long line of nonpregnant, non-child-toting adults, but then again, my feet did hurt from lugging around the extra pounds, and the chair looked mighty appealing. I took the seat gratefully; within minutes I was ushered to the window. No one in the longer line seemed the least bit annoyed.

I soon learned that this was standard practice in every bank, every municipal office—anywhere that there was a line. The joke was that you could earn good money standing outside the bank and "renting out" your baby to people who wanted to use the express line.

Even the airport had separate, shorter lines for pregnant women and families with children. In my seventh month of pregnancy I had to fly back to the United States, alone, for a conference. The minute I entered the departure terminal in San José, an airline employee rushed up and grabbed my bags. He hauled them over to the counter and then escorted me to the front of the line. The same thing happened at the security checkpoint and again when I boarded the plane. It was all so strange, but also so welcoming. I'd never before experienced so many strangers so willing to help without their even being asked.

In the United States, the difference—and indifference—was palpable. In the Pittsburgh airport I used one of the airport carts to carry my heavy bag (I'd packed an overambitious number of books). As I wheeled it toward security, a guard informed me that carts were not allowed in the restricted area. I apologized and told him that I needed the cart because I was unable to carry the bag. As one who'd always had unlimited energy, this wasn't the easiest thing to admit, but I had to face my physical limitations at the moment. I hoped that my very pregnant state would offer a reasonable—and obvious—explanation, and that a dispensation would be offered. He simply shrugged, repeating the injunction that carts were not allowed. While he stood watching, I abandoned the cart and lugged the bag by hand for the last fifty yards.

On the trip back, in the Philadelphia airport, there were a series of delays, and then a last-minute plane switch. I was informed that if I wanted to catch my desired flight to Costa Rica, I'd have to run down the hall—now!—eight gates away, before the plane doors were irrevocably shut. At first I thought the employee was joking, but when I figured out that she wasn't, I hitched my arms under my belly and sprinted. There are aerodynamic reasons, I quickly learned, why pregnant women do not typically participate in the Olympic hundred-yard dash. In my head, I quickly reviewed the mechanics of the placenta and cushioning effects of amniotic fluid as I loped awkwardly down the hall, praying that these biological wonders were indeed as wondrous as the textbooks promised. Not once during my deranged display of athleticism did a single airport employee offer to help.

I arrived at the gate, but the door was already closed. I was breathless, sweaty, and nearly unhinged, but I was determined to get back to my family in Costa Rica. I banged on the door, hollering like a lunatic until a flight attendant opened from the other side. I beseeched her to let me on the flight, and after an inordinately painful pause, she granted admittance. I was so grateful to be going home.

Chapter Fifteen

As my due date approached, we realized that we needed someone who could care for Naava and Noah when labor started—
someone who could commit to a long babysitting stint for which
we could predict neither date nor time nor duration. We'd met a
teacher from Colombia who was in Costa Rica without her family
and so had relative flexibility. She willingly agreed to be our "night
person" should the need arise. The only hitch was that she needed
to be out of town for just one Saturday night, as she was interviewing for a teaching position on the Caribbean coast.

As luck would have it, my contractions began at eleven on that
very Saturday night. I called Dr. Agosín. When I told him about
our babysitter glitch, he said that the hospital wasn't too busy and
that, if we needed to, we could bring our two children and let them
sleep there. By two in the morning, we couldn't wait any longer.
We tucked Naava and Noah into trusty Juan Carlos, thankful that
the hospital was ten minutes away and not two blocks away, like
in New York. Ten minutes in the car at 2:00 a.m. would surely lull
two young children back to sleep.

I had evidently underestimated the power of a two- and four-
year-old to stay awake when they sensed something in the air. I
had also underestimated the painful experience of driving a suspen-
sion-challenged minivan over the Costa Rican cobblestones and
potholes while in labor. We arrived at the hospital with two very
wide-awake children and one very discombobulated mother.

One of the beauties of a small hospital is that it is, well, small.
As I trundled through the door, my condition was fairly obvious—
language skills were unnecessary—and within minutes I was on the
OB floor in a gown, getting settled onto a bed.

The contractions were worsening quickly, and the anesthesiologist was on his way over to place the epidural. I was twisting
and turning, trying vainly to find a comfortable position, when
out of the corner of my eye I caught sight of an image that multi-
plied my anxiety fivefold: walking down the hallway—I saw them
from behind—were Naava and Noah with Benjy between them,

holding their hands. Wearing purple and pink stripy pajamas, Velcro sandals, and matching black hooded sweatshirts, Naava and Noah dragged their identical backpacks filled with toys and books, looking as sweet and innocent and out of place as could be imagined.

I was suddenly jolted by the reality of the situation we'd found ourselves in. It was absolutely wrong that we'd brought a two- and four-year-old to the hospital with us. It would be terrifying for Naava and Noah to see me in this state—writhing, crying, in pain. They wouldn't be able to comprehend what was going on and would be frightened and unsettled.

At that moment, I was overwhelmed by a strange sort of loneliness. We didn't have family here in Costa Rica who could be relied upon unconditionally. We had made friends, but we'd only known them a short time and didn't yet know how large a favor could be asked. We were the newcomers in our community. Despite having reasonable security in many other facets of our lives—financial, political, career, basic health—we were still strangers here.

The unvarnished reality was that we were alone in a hospital in Central America in the middle of the night, with a baby who had no intention of waiting for a more convenient moment, two dazed children who needed to be cared for, right now, and the only Spanish speaker of the family doubled over in pain. There was not a single soul who was going to materialize and say, "I'll take care of this."

Benjy bundled our confused children back into Juan Carlos and drove them home. In the pitch-darkness of the night, he knocked on the door of our neighbors. Despite the fact that we hadn't given them any warning, they were delightfully generous. Barbara bounded out of bed and came to our house in pajamas and slippers. Naava and Noah were a bit whimpery at first, but apparently they settled in fine, listening to hours of German-accented stories until morning.

Meanwhile, my labor was progressing precipitously. I worried that Benjy wouldn't make it back to the hospital in time. The basics of the delivery-room process were similar to those in New York, except for the fact that they took place in Spanish.

"*Cien por ciento borrado,*" Dr. Agosín said to the nurse. "*Diez centímetros dilitado.*"

"*Déme un minuto para el epidural,*" the anesthesiologist said.

The nurse shook her head. "*No tenemos bastante tiempo. Ella está ya en la tercera estación.*"

"*No se preocupe,*" the anesthesiologist said, elbowing her jocularly. "*Soy el más rápido del mundo. Déme treinta segundos entre las contracciones y la alcanzaré.*" He turned to me. "Just tell me when the contraction ends. I'll have the epidural in before you can sneeze."

"*Espere,*" I said. We had to wait.

"*¿Espere?*" the nurse asked me. "*¿Espere en el epidural?*"

"No," I said. I needed that epidural—now—but I wanted to wait for Benjy for the actual delivery, and I knew the nurse didn't speak any English. "*Lo hace…,*" I tried. "*Lo haces…*" What the hell was the imperative form of *to do*?

"*¡Lo haga!*" I said, finally nailing it. "*¡Haga el epidural! Pero…*" Then my confidence faltered. "*…Espere por mi esposo.*" Or was it *espere para mi esposo*? I'd never mastered the distinction between *por* and *para*.

"Don't worry," Dr. Agosín said to me in English. "I won't break your water until your husband arrives."

Suddenly I was flooded with the compulsion to push. "I don't think…," I started. "*Yo no sé…*" And then I spied Benjy at the door, stuffing his six-foot frame into size-small scrubs, the only pair handy. He hustled in just as baby Ariel pushed her 3,600 grams into the earliest flickers of a Costa Rican sunrise.

"*El Apgar es nueve en un minuto,*" Dr. Agosín said calmly to the nurse. "*Diez en cinco minutos.*"

After that, I tuned out the conversation. There was simply no energy left to translate. I'd have to make do without keeping tabs on the medical banter. I would just have to be a patient.

I expected Dr. Agosín and the anesthesiologist to exit within five minutes, as I recalled the usual procedure in New York, leaving me with the nurses for the prolonged cleanup. But they didn't leave. At first I thought maybe there'd been a complication that they weren't telling me about.

But that wasn't the case. Dr. Agosín and the anesthesiologist stayed for almost an hour, doing all the cleanup themselves. They helped me with the baby, adjusting her to lie comfortably on my chest. They didn't seem in any sort of rush. When I expressed my surprise at this, both doctors laughed. "This is the best part," Dr. Agosín said. "All the tensions are gone and now we can relax and enjoy the new baby with you."

I slept for a few hours in my hospital room, then awoke, ravenous for food but even more ravenous for a shower. Esperanza—a trim nurse in her late twenties—handed me a package of toiletries and gestured me to the shower. An older, stouter nurse aide named Zenelia arrived with towels. The two of them stood outside the door while I showered, just in case I needed help. This contrasted starkly with my experience in New York, where I'd been handed a plastic squeeze bottle and left to fend for myself. I'd limped down the hall to a lone shower stall, hoping the call button inside worked despite the running water.

Now, with Esperanza and Zenelia standing discreetly outside the shower door, I felt safe and reassured. The steaming water washed away the sticky remnants of the delivery and eased the aching fatigue. The steam accumulated, creating a soothing cloud of warmth around my body. I could feel my muscles thaw, one by one, in the delicious heat. The wooziness was luscious, tempting, and my anxiety began to seep away. Soon it was my consciousness that began to seep away. As my blood pressure plummeted and I began to faint, I suddenly found myself swooped into the arms of two women, then lowered gently to the floor. Zenelia wrapped me in towels and Esperanza waved smelling salts under my nose.

As I came back to life, I tried to right myself, but they shushed me, imploring me to rest. *"Descansa, mi amor, descansa,"* Zenelia said while Esperanza maneuvered in her sphygmomanometer to check my blood pressure.

After ten minutes, my blood pressure rose to normal levels, and my mind gradually began to clear. My hair was still packed with shampoo, as I'd passed out before I'd been able to rinse. I tried to explain that I needed to get back into the shower to rinse it out. *"No, no."* They shook their heads, clucking. *"Nosotros lo hacemos."*

Zenelia brought a plastic basin from under the sink and tipped my head back over it, supporting my head with her sturdy right hand. Esperanza poured cupfuls of warm water over my hair, and the two of them worked their fingers through my scalp and hair. They took their time, working each strand from root to tip. My muscles were completely lax; my body was enveloped in their arms and their quiet murmurings in Spanish. I couldn't follow a word of what they were saying, but it didn't matter. I felt so completely cared for, in a way that I'd never before experienced as an adult. Certainly never in my two prior experiences of giving birth.

A few hours later, Benjy arrived with Naava and Noah in tow. The children had spent the entire night awake listening to Barbara's stories, so this ten-minute car ride accomplished what the last one had failed to—both kids were fast asleep when they arrived at the hospital. Benjy parked their car seats in the corner of the room, where they slept for hours. Ariel was curled in the crook of my arm in a postprandial haze. I was still under the lingering euphoric effects of Esperanza's and Zenelia's ministrations. Benjy took one look at the daybed under the windowsill—simple, but horizontal— and stretched out, promptly dropping off to sleep.

I gazed at my family, each person asleep in one position or another, happy that all were comfortable and together, finally able to relax after the roller coaster of the last twenty-four hours. We had survived the biggest hurdle of the year, and now we could rest.

After napping well into the afternoon, Naava and Noah finally awoke. They were excited to see their new baby sister but were frankly more eager to explore this new place. They examined every shelf, drawer, and corner of my room. They investigated the corridor, the ward, the elevators, and the lobby. Nobody seemed to mind two kids scampering about.

When my dinner arrived, I was surprised to see that there was also a meal for Benjy, though by now I was becoming accustomed to this attitude. The two dinner trays—arranged nicely on a bedside table that had a white sheet draped over it—were without a doubt the highlight of the entire birth experience for Naava and Noah. They scarfed down the soup, the *arroz con pollo,* and the plantains, occasionally holding out spoonfuls for us. Not one staff member said anything about visiting hours being over or that children were not permitted. Only when Naava and Noah had scraped away the last of the *tres leches* was it clear that they were ready for bed.

Having a new baby opened up another layer of Costa Rican society for me. A week after Ariel was born, we returned to the hospital for our first pediatrician visit. After the visit, I sat with Ariel on the hospital steps, waiting for Benjy to bring Juan Carlos around. In those few minutes, no fewer than thirty strangers stopped to admire the baby, offer congratulations, ask after my health, even bless the baby.

Two months later, we were in a restaurant when Ariel vocally announced her need for a clean diaper. The pitch of crying and the attendant discomfort made it evident that our meal could not progress until this matter was addressed. I gathered our supplies and headed toward the public bathroom, hoping there was some sort of counter or that the floor wasn't too dirty. As I crossed the restaurant, the owner darted out from behind the register and directed me to the back door of the restaurant. Before I could say a word, we were out the door, walking into her home behind the restaurant. She led me to her bedroom, laid out a fresh towel on her bed, and helped me arrange baby and supplies in a clean, comfortable setting.

A few weeks later I walked into a small souvenir store, stacked to the rafters with the wooden handicrafts that Costa Rica is known for. I balanced Ariel against my left shoulder as I poked through a stack of wooden salad bowls. Then I shifted her to my right shoulder as I examined the wooden toys. The proprietor walked up to me and offered to hold the baby while I shopped. I couldn't imagine such an offer in New York, nor could I have ever imagined acceding. Yet it seemed perfectly natural here. I handed Ariel off to a perfect stranger and shopped while the two of them entertained each other.

Over and over—in stores, hotels, restaurants, markets—Ticos offered to hold my baby and seemed to delight in it. This became standard operating procedure in my day-to-day life with Ariel, and

I quickly appreciated how much easier it was to travel with a baby when there was such a vast "extended family" available and happy to help. Suddenly, I was meeting people from all walks of life. I was having conversations with people I'd never otherwise have engaged with. If I ever had another baby, I thought, I would surely do it in Costa Rica.

⸺⊗⊗⊗⸺

The year in Costa Rica was a wonderful respite from the high-octane pace of New York City. Naava and Noah picked up an impressive amount of Spanish. They learned how to ride bicycles over cobblestones and through potholes. They learned the best technique for lobbing a *limón dulce* at one's sibling. They learned the pleasures of playing in the drenching afternoon rains, soaking themselves through and through, knowing that a late-day sun would eventually pop out. They learned that fresh coconuts chopped open by machete offered a free sweet drink. They learned that school was much more fun when rabbits, chickens, squirrels, and a lumbering sow resided in the backyard. They grew accustomed to social gatherings at which twelve different languages were spoken. Ariel spent her first six months being passed happily from hand to hand, cooed over, rocked, and sung to. There was only one lullaby in Costa Rica, it seemed, perhaps just one in all of Latin America—"*Los Pollitos.*" To this day, it remains Ariel's favorite song.

⸺⊗⊗⊗⸺

When the year was over, we reluctantly packed our bags and said good-bye to our friends and neighbors, who had grown to be part of an extended family for us. I knew it would be a difficult transition to leave this society, but I hadn't imagined it would be so abrupt. When we landed in Miami three hours after our tearful good-byes in Escazú, the airline workers refused to unload the strollers and wheelchairs from the plane until all the other customers had left. The elderly, the infirm, and the families with young children sat just inside the terminal, watching everyone else march off the plane.

The next plane landed and unloaded its customers. Finally, after nearly an hour, the strollers and wheelchairs appeared. By the time we'd made it through passport control, gathered our eleven suitcases, and dragged our entourage from international arrivals to domestic departures, our connecting flight had left without us. That 11:00 p.m. flight was the last plane to New York City that day.

"Next flight's at six thirty a.m. tomorrow," the American Airlines agent said. "I suggest you get some rest and come to the ticket counter at five a.m." He gestured to the floor of the waiting lounge, where other stranded travelers were beginning to settle down for the night.

"You can't be serious, sir," I said. "I have three little children, including a six-month-old baby."

He shrugged and gave a half-sympathetic smile. "There's nothing we can do, ma'am. I could give you a restaurant coupon, but all the restaurants are closed now."

Realizing that we had no other options, we arranged our suitcases in a circle, sort of like the pioneers of the West circling their wagons. In the next group over, a pregnant woman struggled to get comfortable on the floor. We unearthed the remaining snacks in our carry-ons and distributed them to the children. Their fatigue caused them to shiver uncontrollably, so we pulled towels out of the suitcases and wrapped them up like mummies. Their faces were expressionless by now—wan and defeated—and their bodies without resistance as we tucked them into a makeshift bed of jackets and towels, pushing them close together for body heat.

Benjy and I each took turns staying awake to keep an eye on our possessions while the other one slept with the children. As I curled myself around baby Ariel, my arms stretched over Naava and Noah, one thought trailed through my head: this would never happen in Costa Rica. If pregnant women and families with babies were stuck overnight in the airport, sleeping on the floor, the employees would have immediately invited the passengers to their own homes. I had no doubt about it. I lay my head against the stiff carpet and wished I could will us back to Costa Rica for just one more night.

When we finally landed in New York the next day, my eyes cringed at the overwhelming concrete and the near utter absence of green. But still, my heart fluttered when the taxi pulled up to our building.

I'd been so concerned that the kids would soon forget Costa Rica that I'd stocked up on as many mementos and Spanish storybooks as I could possibly carry. What I hadn't counted on was that they'd forget New York. This was especially the case for Noah. When we opened the door to our apartment he looked around, not recognizing anything. The first thing he asked was "Is there a bathroom here?" It dawned on me that one-third of his entire life had been spent in Costa Rica and, at this moment, it was the only existence that he was aware of.

I brought him to his bedroom, and he spied a stuffed frog that had been a special toy of his. His eyes lit up and then he said, "Oh, let's take this one home."

"We *are* home, Noah," I told him gently.

"No, I mean home in Costa Rica," he said with a pleading look in his eyes.

And that's how it seemed to settle in him, and in us as well. It was as though we had two homes, even if everything from our life in Costa Rica was now gone. We'd even managed to sell our van, though for a solid year Noah's eyes welled up with tears at the merest mention of Juan Carlos.

The country that had initially been so foreign to us had now taken on aspects of home. There was a special sense of calm that I associated with Costa Rica that filled a certain spot in my heart. Whenever I experienced episodes similar to our night on the floor of the Miami airport, I yearned for the home of Costa Rica.

Perhaps this was how immigrants eventually found peace with their adopted countries, by somehow finding spots in their hearts for their new and old homes. Naava and Noah would always have an association with a year of freedom, so different from the more restricted life in New York City, not to mention their perfectly accented Spanish and fondness for *limón dulce*. Benjy and I would always have an association with this break from our regular lives, with this year of slow-paced living filled with new friends and abundant luscious fruits.

But of course it is the one who retained no recollections of Costa Rica whatsoever—my daughter Ariel—who would actually carry a solid bit of it forever. Her American passport listed Escazú, Costa Rica, as the place of birth (with no mention, however, of living three hundred meters south of the *supermercado*). I didn't know if she would choose to continue dual citizenship as an adult, but for now there was a República de Costa Rica passport with a grinning baby, bald as a saucer, ears spread wide like satellite dishes. Nationality: *Costarricense.*

Part Three

✎ Chapter Sixteen ✎

Returning to Bellevue after a year away was a peculiar sensation. In most ways, everything was just as I'd left it. My colleagues were still in their same windowless offices, seeing the same patients with diabetes and hypertension, battling the same irritating computer system. The same skirmishes with administrators over staffing, supplies, and scheduling were still going on. The same annoyances about "productivity" and "efficiency" were still being bandied about.

But I felt different. I felt well rested in a way that I hadn't felt in years. In Costa Rica there had been a palpable absence of tension. I described it to a friend, saying that in New York we always had twenty-seven balls in the air, but in Costa Rica, there were no balls at all. For a classic type-A personality, I was surprised at how much the life of leisure suited me. We'd always heard those stories about people who went on vacations to other countries and then never came back. I now understood how easily that could happen.

This rested feeling stayed with me, at least for a while. As I re-entered the medical world, I could feel the frenzy bearing down on that warm spot of Costa Rican tranquillity that I fought to hang on to. It became increasingly beleaguered, however, as the realities of New York City, Bellevue, and American life set in.

Julia Barquero was one of the first patients I saw when I returned. She had become my regular patient shortly after we'd first met in the hospital, after the resident who was her clinic doctor—the one who had finally given her the grim news about her prognosis—had graduated, as had the cardiology fellow. I was the only one who had known her from the beginning, so her care drifted into my hands. Julia turned out to be a wonderful patient. She was organized and reliable. She kept track of her complex and changing pill regimen as well as of her many clinic appointments.

The first thing I noticed when she walked into the office was how wonderful she looked—healthy, robust. When I'd met her in the hospital ward, I assumed she'd be dead or severely disabled within a few years; after all, that's what the studies on people with such weakened hearts showed. But those studies could only report on what happened to the population on average, not to the individual.

In fact, Julia was outperforming the data. With her daily allotment of pills, her resilient body compensated beautifully. She did not have swollen legs or fluid-laden lungs. She had sufficient energy to walk up and down the three flights of stairs to her apartment. Her clinic visits that followed her initial hospitalization had been pro forma—merely renewing her prescriptions, checking in on how she was doing.

The issue of the heart transplant never came up again in conversation, but it was an underlying *basso continuo*—at least in *my* head—during all of our encounters. Whenever I read in the newspaper about the latest crackdown on illegal immigrants, there was always the requisite diatribe about immigrants taking advantage of the American health-care system. I wasn't a nativist, but I had to admit that I could see their point. Shortly after one of my closest friends died at age twenty-seven of a congenital cardiomyopathy, his father had needed a heart transplant for the identical condition. If he'd died while waiting on the list while a heart had gone to an undocumented immigrant, I would have been furious at the injustice.

Of course, Julia Barquero wasn't any random undocumented immigrant; she was the real person sitting in front of me, the patient I was caring for. *Of course* she deserved a heart transplant, for the simple reason that she was going to die without one. This conclusion was patently obvious to me. It was simply ethically just.

But we always told our interns not to practice medicine by anecdote. Wouldn't this simply be practicing ethics by anecdote? Why should Julia Barquero merit a heart just because she was sitting here in my office, just because she'd been successful in sneaking into this country illegally?

I winced at these thoughts as they needled below the surface during our clinic visits. Julia never expressed anger or sadness about her medical condition. She never asked me any further questions about prognosis. She never pressed me for details.

Today felt like a reunion as we caught up on the past year. Lucita had started preschool and was thriving. Julia's husband was still in Florida doing the roofing jobs under the broiling sun that no one else wanted, but this enabled them to send small sums of money back to the family in Guatemala. I recalled that Julia's son, Vasco, was being raised by her mother, and I was sure that this extra money was crucial.

Before I could start down my list of cardiac questions, Julia pulled out a white, hand-knitted baby cap from her bag and pressed it toward me. *"Para su bebé—la Tica."* Inside the cap was a card that contained a neatly folded five-dollar bill. I tried to demur on the money, but Julia would have none of it. *"Para su bebé,"* she repeated.

She climbed onto the exam table and I traced my stethoscope along the quadrants of her lungs. I was rewarded with the smooth sibilance of unhindered respiration, no crackles or rales suggestive of fluid retention. The jugular veins in her neck—the body's natural manometers that bulged like pulsing serpents when cardiac pressures rose—were beautifully flat.

"¿Cómo está Vasco?" I asked as I bent down to palpate her calves, noting the complete absence of edema.

Julia paused and slowly brought her hands to her brow. *"No está bien,"* she said.

I stopped my exam and straightened up. *"¿No está bien?"* I asked.

Julia began telling me a complicated story about Vasco and *fronteras.* Now was the time for my improved Spanish to kick in, but then she said something about *en cárcel* and I really became confused. I knew that *cárcel* meant "jail," but Vasco was eight years old, so there was something I was missing. Despite Rigoberto's weekly drills on idioms and his insistence on Spanish as it had been spoken by Cervantes, I was still having trouble. How could a story about an eight-year-old involve jail?

Painstakingly I chipped away at the Spanish version of the story, reassembling the fragments in English. Indeed her son was being held in a detention center. Julia and her husband had saved forty-five hundred dollars to pay a coyote to bring Vasco to America. Vasco and the coyote had been running in the desert, across the Texan border, in the dead of night when Vasco's shoe became loose.

He stumbled, then simply plopped onto the ground, unable or un-willing to go forward. The coyote, who didn't want to get caught, ran off, leaving the boy alone. Eventually both Vasco and the coyote were picked up by border police. Vasco had been instructed by the coyote to use a false name, one that had been selected to help him get over the border. But he couldn't—maybe it was his learning dis-ability, Julia thought. The coyote was deported, but because Vasco was a minor, he was being held at a detention center in Texas.

I curled my stethoscope into my pocket as Julia slipped off the exam table and sank into the chair.

"I want to see him so badly," she said in Spanish, eyes weighted with desperation, "but they say it can take weeks. I'm too scared to be away from Bellevue for so long. What if something happens?"

"Have they said what they will do with him?" I asked.

She shook her head in slow motion. "If he is deported back to Guatemala, this might be my only chance to see him. I'm so scared." She pulled the edges of her lavender sweater tighter around her nar-row shoulders. "Maybe you could write a letter about my medical condition? Maybe that would help?"

I typed a letter while Julia sat hunched in her chair, sniffling oc-casionally. I documented her severely weakened heart. I listed the panoply of medications she was taking. I commented on the "grave prognosis." I printed it out and handed it to her.

I wished I could imbue the sheet of paper with real powers. I wished I could will a new heart for Julia, an easy reunion with Vasco. Why did it all have to be so fraught? Why did this one person have to suffer so much? Why did this perfectly ordinary woman have to face imminent death *and* worry about never seeing her child again?

A guilty pang of regret for leaving Costa Rica sneaked in at that moment. Would that life could have stayed so simple, that the deepest worry could be whether the consuming dampness of the rainy season would warp the wood of a cello or whether the kids had applied enough sunscreen to ward off the tropical sun…

We stood up to say good-bye. Once again I tried to pass the five-dollar bill back to Julia. She refused to take it.

❧ Chapter Seventeen ❧

Three weeks later, my clinic roster was crammed again. The morning session overflowed into my afternoon session, and any hope for getting lunch evaporated. When I'd taken Juliet out on her early-morning walk that day, I'd noticed the first fingerlings of autumn crispness in the air and I'd been hoping to grab a few minutes at lunchtime to sneak outside for a quick dose. Instead I pulled out my yogurt and stirred it up while finishing the morning charts. Two minutes later I realized that I'd slurped down the entire container and couldn't even recall what flavor it was.

A vivid memory of a spontaneous block party in Costa Rica came to mind. I'd cooked up a huge vat of vegetable soup for our dinner one evening, more than we could possibly eat. When I spied our next-door neighbors walking back from the market, I beckoned them over for a bowl. Then I saw the family from Holland returning from school and I called to them to help us out. Word got around the neighborhood, and someone showed up with a bottle of wine, someone else with empanadas, another person with *gallo pinto*. Soon our veranda was filled with food, drink, and conversation while an azure twilight settled around us. The scent of hibiscus flowers—always especially potent after the daily rain—floated like a fragrant fog over everyone.

A sharp knock on my door interrupted my thoughts. The medical assistant popped her head in and reminded me, apologetically, that there were three charts in the box, and two patients were already complaining about the wait. "Oh, and here are the phone messages and med refills that backed up from the morning," she added, pressing a stack of papers into my hand.

I grabbed the pile of messages from yesterday with my other hand and waved them in her face. "And what about these?" I snapped. "When am I supposed to finish the ones from yesterday?" I slammed them all onto my desk as the assistant hurriedly pulled the door closed.

It's gone, I thought, sinking my head into my arms atop the sea of paper debris. Every last bit of calm and peacefulness from that year of repose was gone. Extirpated by the insanity of this life and this job. I thought about that spontaneous gathering of friends in Costa Rica. In Manhattan, we could never host a party like that because our apartment's size allowed only two guests at a time—and they had to be on very good terms with each other. The veranda in Costa Rica, by contrast, was a seemingly infinite space; neighbors easily spilled over onto the yard, the kids climbed on the rocks or scampered to the playground.

But the starker contrast was that of time: Somehow people seemed to have time for a spontaneous party. Nobody was rushed. Such an event could never have happened in New York, even with my closest and dearest friends. Everyone's life here was scheduled so tightly. What were we all so busy with?

The medical assistant knocked again, this time more gingerly. "Dr. Ofri," she said, nearly in a whisper, "your next patient is here."

Mohammed Khalil limped slightly, his body canting to the right as he entered the room. He grasped the edge of my desk and lowered himself into the chair, extending his left leg straight ahead while the right was comfortably bent. He was fifty-four, compact but rotund, with a pulvinate belly that settled comfortably on his thighs. He wore a brightly patterned embroidered vest over his button-down shirt; a matching embroidered cap was perched on his crown.

Despite his obvious discomfort, he smiled broadly at me when I introduced myself. Two gold teeth glittered, framed by a neatly trimmed gray beard and mustache.

"I have torn the medical meniscus," he told me, tripping over the term in his moderately accented English. "They did MRI for me in New Jersey," he added, pressing a large manila envelope into my hands, "and maybe I must have surgery."

I took a deep breath. "Tell me what's been going on with your knee," I said, shoving the stack of messages to the far corner of my desk and then easing the films out of the envelope.

"Well, as you see, I have trouble to bend." He pointed to the left knee. "It hurts too much, so I need to keep straight mostly."

The decision to surgically repair a torn medial meniscus depended on a person's physical condition and needs. Most surgeons would repair a meniscus in a young person who would be physically active for many decades. For an elderly, sedentary person, conservative management with physical therapy was preferable. For a middle-aged person at the center of the spectrum, one needed to get a sense of his or her life and how physical it was.

"How much bending do you generally do?" I asked.

Mr. Khalil chuckled when I asked this. "Five times a day I have to kneel for prayer," he said, circling his hands in the air for emphasis. "It's not so easy!"

"Is there any possibility of sitting in a chair, rather than kneeling? Are there exceptions made for illness?"

"But I am imam," he said, amused at my ignorance. "I must set example." He went on to tell me that he led a mosque in Queens. He'd moved from Iraq with his wife and five children two decades ago and set up shop in a mosque in Flushing, just underneath the number 7 subway. On the exam table he rolled up his pants and extended his legs for me to examine. I palpated the knee joints on both sides. The right one was certainly more tender, but there was no joint instability or any signs of acute inflammation. I could hear crepitus as I flexed and extended each knee—the crinkling-newspaper sound of bone rubbing against bone, suggesting worn-away cartilage. I would refer him to the orthopedists to weigh the risks and benefits of surgery, but I'd definitely encourage physical therapy in the meanwhile.

Back at the desk, I coaxed the MRI scans back into the envelope and then handed it back to Mr. Khalil, and he tucked it inside an Arabic newspaper. As I wrote out the referral to orthopedics, I noticed him scanning the headlines.

"What's in the news?" I asked.

All the cheeriness drained from Mr. Khalil's face. "Bad news," he said in a pained voice. "Always bad news."

It had been more than five years since the United States had invaded Iraq. Sectarian violence waxed and waned but never seemed to stop. American deaths had topped four thousand, and Iraqi deaths were in the tens of thousands.

"Have you lost anyone in the war?" I asked softly.

"Everyone has lost someone in war," he said, his face tightening awkwardly. "Two friends killed by car bomb last month shopping in market—shopping! It's way of life now."

Mr. Khalil fingered the edges of the MRI envelope with his chipped nails. "But now is no worse than before. In 1982, my three brothers arrested by Saddam Hussein—twenty-two, eighteen, and littlest one four years old. We never saw them again." He leaned down and stuffed the MRI envelope and newspaper into the bag next to his chair. "After war started and records released, we learned what happened. Buried alive—all three of them. Even the little boy." He paused. "Sometimes better not to know."

Then he looked up at me, seeming to want to change the subject. "You? Where are you from?"

I told him that on my father's side my grandparents were from Yemen and my father had been raised in Israel. My mother's family was from Eastern Europe.

"So you are Jewish?" His voice was polite, inquisitive, devoid of any of the bitterness from a few moments ago.

I found myself hesitating before this question, uncomfortable with my own unease. As a rule, I did not discuss my religion, or anything about myself, for that matter. If a patient asked, and I didn't think the information would interfere with our primary goal of his health, then I'd answer honestly but wouldn't necessarily elaborate.

With Mr. Khalil I wasn't sure. Would this introduce a political element to our relationship? Would a discussion of Middle East politics supersede the one about his medial meniscus? Would we soon be debating about East Jerusalem, Hamas, and Gaza? Would the conversation unearth simmering historical arguments over Tel Chai and Deir Yassin? I didn't have the time or the energy or the desire for this sort of thing.

My Hispanic patients were all probably aware that I was Jewish because they'd been coming to Bellevue for generations and knew that half the doctors disappeared on Rosh Hashanah and Yom Kippur. But they rarely asked. It seemed it was only my Muslim patients who asked, and always—like Mr. Khalil—politely, directly, and with genuine curiosity. I did not get the sense that Mr. Khalil was here to argue politics. I did not think religious differences would adversely affect our relationship, though in today's polarized world, I supposed, there was always that slight risk.

But then I chided myself for my hesitation. We were in Manhattan, not Riyadh or Hebron. "Yes," I replied to Mr. Khalil, "I am Jewish."

The warm smile returned to his face. "Muslim and Jews; we are brothers. And you are Arab Jew." His forthcoming nature drove home to me how unfounded my concerns were. I was glad that we lived in New York—though I might have preferred Costa Rica on a day like this—and were able to connect in ways that would probably not be possible in the Middle East.

Mr. Khalil and I stood up. I felt very simpatico with him and held out my hand to say good-bye. *"Salaam aleikum,"* I said, using the only Arabic that I knew.

"Aleikum salaam," he replied, clearly delighted. But he immediately pulled his hand out of my reach. He lowered his voice. "You understand, right?"

I nodded my head, though actually I was not quite sure I did. Would he not shake my hand because I was a woman or because I was a Jew or because he was paranoid about infections? I was familiar enough with ultra Orthodox Jews, though, to suspect that it was a parallel religious prohibition against touching women. I didn't press the issue or even ask why he'd allowed me to examine his knee if my touch was forbidden.

At least there was that commonality in our religions, I noted ironically: similar taboos about women. Perhaps that could be the starting point of mutuality in the next round of Arab-Israeli peace talks!

Mr. Khalil limped out of my office, and I bade him a speedy recovery.

—⁂—

My next three patients were a blur to me. Ana Velez, Milagros Santana, and Reina Rodriguez—sweet middle-aged ladies—all spoke Dominican Spanish at Mach-3 velocity. They grappled with diabetes, hypertension, weight, and cholesterol, plus a smattering of osteoporosis, dyspepsia, and hypothyroidism, but it was the so-cial stresses that made their medical care so challenging.

Mrs. Santana had been raising her two teenage grandchildren since her daughter had died of AIDS; the younger of the two had also been infected with HIV. Mrs. Velez's husband had been inca-pacitated by a stroke, and she had to attend to his prodigious medi-cal needs. Mrs. Rodriguez's finances were always on the brink, no matter how many jobs she worked, because she was always send-ing money to family back home.

They were salt-of-the-urban-earth women, suffering the aches and pains from working as housekeepers and babysitters, sagging under the weight of being the fulcrums of their families.

None had space or time for friends or hobbies—there was only work and taking care of family. Whenever I asked about support systems, the answer was never *husband, friends, coworkers, rela-tives, neighbors*. The answer was always the same—*la iglesia*. Mrs. Velez rose at 5:00 a.m. to attend an early service before her hus-band awoke. Mrs. Santana had one prayer only for Jesus: that he would keep her grandchildren away from the drugs that had ruined her daughter and would also quickly invent a cure for AIDS. Mrs. Rodriguez could only duck into the church near her subway stop for a few minutes between jobs. It was a Korean church now, but it sufficed.

———— ⌘ ————

Efrain Jimenez was a whole other story. He bustled into my office, apologized for being late—even though I was later than he was—and flopped into the chair. With a soft, dimpled face and narrow eyes, he looked much younger than sixty-five. His fluid extra chin curved smoothly from either side of his frizzy gray goatee. Today he wore a black silk Chinese suit—loose boxy jacket with elaborate woven buttons and baggy drawstring pants. A black wool fishing cap sat evenly on the center of his nearly bald head.

"How are you today, Mr. Jimenez?" I asked, glancing at the clock, thinking that I would never get through this day.

He turned up his palms and arms in a distinctly Eastern European manner and said, "*Baruch Hashem*, at least I am alive."

Mr. Jimenez looked and sounded like a Puerto Rican version of Tevye the dairyman from *Fiddler on the Roof*. The first time we'd met, he leaned in close to me and asked sotto voce, "You're a member of the tribe, Doctor, aren't you?"

When I nodded, the whole story came pouring out. Raised in the Bronx, a self-described mongrel—his mother was Puerto Rican Catholic from a Basque family who spoke to him in Spanish, his father a mix of Native American and African American who spoke to him in Italian—Mr. Jimenez converted to Judaism when he married a Jewish woman, approaching religion with a convert's zeal. His children—Rivka, Moishe, and Yitzhak—attended Jewish day schools. Though his wife had divorced him many years ago and had since died of cancer, Mr. Jimenez still identified himself as Jewish.

"I don't belong to a shul now—I'm embarrassed to say—but who can afford the memberships these days," he said, waving his fleshy hands in the air. "It's all meshuga. But even if I'm lapsed, Hashem still knows the goodness of a soul."

He was proud that Rivka had remained Orthodox, living in Borough Park, Brooklyn, keeping kosher. "Such a beauty. Smart too—a real *yiddishe kop* she has. Now if she'd only find a nice Jewish doctor. You'd think there'd be a million of them in New York..."

Today, Mr. Jimenez announced to me that he'd completely stopped using marijuana for the past two months. "No brownies, no joints, no nothing. And no meat. I've given up red meat altogether. My only vice"—he looked me in the eye to check for approval or disapproval—"is dark chocolate. I eat exactly one square of dark chocolate every night before bed. They say that the antioxidants are miraculous, but only if you get the good stuff from South America. None of this Hershey's dreck."

I gathered the energy to congratulate Mr. Jimenez on his accomplishments, but reminded him that chocolate—even the antioxidant-laden dark kind—wasn't so good for his diabetes. "Sugar is sugar," I said, "and yours hasn't dipped into the normal range in a couple of years. We may have to start insulin to control it."

Mr. Jimenez held up his hands in a mock cross to ward off the insulin vampire. "I'm not taking insulin. I will get my sugar under control, I promise. I know that beets are really helpful. All I have to do is get that damn juicer fixed, and then you'll see my sugar come way down."

As I worked on renewing his prescriptions, Mr. Jimenez pointed to the picture of my children. *"Kein ayin hara,"* he said, using the Yiddish phrase that traditionally wards off the evil eye that might jinx a compliment. "Your children are beautiful. *Kein ayin hara,* they'll grow up healthy and strong. I hope you are giving them a good Jewish education."

I nodded my head vaguely as I spread the ten prescriptions on my desk and started signing and stamping them.

"You're doing Jewish day schools, no?" he asked. "The Solomon Schechter schools are excellent. Or are you just doing after-school Hebrew lessons?"

I kept my head down, focused on the prescriptions. I didn't really want to get into a discussion about what—if any—religious education we were choosing for our children, especially because we'd been dancing around that very question for the last few years, and even more especially because there were more patients waiting and this was neither the time nor the place for a Talmudic disquisition.

True to the tribe, Mr. Jimenez kept up the conversation even without me. "Really, the best thing is a yeshiva. Even if yourself aren't religious, it's still best for the kids to get the most traditional education."

My husband, Benjy, had grown up in a modern Orthodox family, attending a religious day school from kindergarten through high school. He was well versed in the rituals and culture, and these aspects remained important to him even as he chose to be less religious during adulthood.

I, on the other hand, had attended public school. I never went to after-school Hebrew lessons but instead spent summers at a socialist Zionist camp in the Catskills debating Marx, Herzl, and Ber Borochov. My father was traditional—attending synagogue every Saturday, keeping a kosher home—but he was mainly alone in this. My mother felt culturally connected to Judaism but not religiously.

Things changed when I started college and my parents moved to

Israel. In Israel—unlike America—it was inconceivable to be neutral on either religion or politics; these issues were crucial matters of the public sphere with palpable consequences. My mother discovered that she was a God-fearing atheist and an ardent left-winger. My father was a Likud supporter, and he grew more religious now that he was "home." Unsurprisingly, my attitudes toward Judaism were complicated to sort out.

"Do you know that I once ran a *cheder*," Mr. Jimenez went on while I finished the prescriptions and prepared an updated medication list for him. *Cheder* is the term for a small religious school, typically for the very orthodox. "Before we had kids, Rachel and I moved out to Wyoming to work near an Indian reservation. Rachel was working in the social service department, and there were a few other Jewish families living out there doing the same sort of thing." Mr. Jimenez's voice grew vibrant as he embroidered his monologue. "I looked around and saw that there was no religious education for these beautiful Jewish children. The nearest shul? Three hundred miles away! It was a shame, a complete *shandeh!*" His palms landed on his thighs with an audible slap. "So what to do? I start a *cheder* myself. Could you imagine, Dr. Ofri? A fat Puerto Rican boy from the Bronx running a *cheder* in Wyoming?" He gave another Tevye-like shrug. "I just hope Hashem appreciated the mitzvah."

I continued to attend to the paperwork, nodding as Mr. Jimenez expanded his story. My years in a Zionist youth group had left me with strong attachments to the cultural aspects of Judaism and Israel. I certainly wanted my children to have a Jewish identity, yet I had trouble relating to a literal interpretation of God.

Benjy and I had visited a number of synagogues in our neighborhood. On the one hand, I found that I couldn't identify with the departures from tradition in the Reform congregations. On the other hand, I couldn't countenance raising my children in an Orthodox synagogue that relegated women behind a screen or up in a distant balcony, no matter how many modern rationalizations were presented. Conservative synagogues seemed like a reasonable compromise, but the formal cantorial style felt distant.

It was a strange sensation to feel so strongly Jewish—enough to want to imbue this in my children—yet be unable to find any sort of communal institution that resonated with me.

In the end, we found an unlikely home—the Tot Shabbat classes in a chilly synagogue basement. The adult service upstairs on Saturday morning was standard issue—reserved, well-meaning, seemingly interminable. Down in the basement, however, parents and kids were singing songs at the top of their lungs, banging on the table to keep the rhythm, playing circle games, telling stories—reveling in the energetic atmosphere, comfortable in jeans and sneakers. It was playful, relaxed, but impressively engaging. The kids learned plenty of prayers and traditions, and the parents enjoyed a Jewish community that was warm, inviting, and—let's face it—fun! It was the unspoken feeling that none of us ever wanted to grow up and have to sit through the adult service upstairs; the children's group was the best place to be.

But I wasn't about to share all this with Mr. Jimenez, as he plainly had definite opinions and I was desperately short on time. I handed him his prescriptions and reminded him about the importance of getting his sugar down, about losing weight, about insulin on the horizon.

"Yeah, yeah, yeah," he said, straightening the cap on his head, brushing off all my words. "I appreciate all you are doing, but you can't change an old *alte cocker* like me. Maybe when the Moshiach comes, I'll be skinny with perfect sugar, but for now, I'll stick with beets and dark chocolate. The good kind. In any case, Yom Kippur is next week and I'll fast for most of the day. That'll knock my sugar down."

Rezual Sarkhel had been pacing in the waiting room for most of the afternoon. He shot me an apprehensive look when I signaled that it was his turn. His taxi shift started in thirty minutes and he couldn't be late. I mumbled my apology, realizing that it had become my reflexive greeting to every patient. As we walked from the waiting room to my office, I slipped a cough drop into my mouth. The menthol was disgusting, but I figured the shot of sugar might help clear my brain.

Mr. Sarkhel bobbed in his chair, even after he was seated, clearly anxious to get out as soon as possible. A fifty-five-year-old Bangladeshi, he'd been in America more than twenty-five years, long enough—we both noted—to acquire an American potbelly.

"It's the taxi driving," he said in his defense. "We only exercise the one foot on the gas pedal and the one finger on the cell phone—that's it. And we always have the food on the front seat next to us, so what do you expect?"

His blood pressure was still not completely controlled, despite three medications. Today, as at every visit for the past year, I was on the verge of starting a fourth medication.

Mr. Sarkhel held up his hands in protest—cell phone gripped in the left. "No, not this time. I promise I'll get rid of the belly. Anyway, Ramadan is coming soon and I'll be fasting every day for a whole month."

"But what about the feasting every night at sunset?"

Mr. Sarkhel stopped bobbing for a moment and hung his head, conceding the point.

"I know what those Middle Eastern desserts are like," I said, pressing onward, "fried in oil, dripping in honey, loaded with enough sugar to rot your teeth on the spot."

"Okay, okay, you got me there," Mr. Sarkhel said. "My wife, she loves to cook sweets. And me, well, I love my wife, so what do I do? I eat all her sweets." He stood up from his chair. "But this Ramadan I will do more fasting than feasting. You'll see," he said, shaking his cell phone for emphasis, "I'll look like a teenager after the month of Ramadan."

I refilled the three hypertension prescriptions and handed them to Mr. Sarkhel, who was already halfway out the door. His phone was ringing and he managed to flick it open with one finger while cramming the prescriptions in his pocket.

The last patient of this seemingly endless afternoon was a thirty-year-old woman named Nazira Houwari. She was tall, regal, and clad in a white silk suit; her heels clicked rhythmically as she entered my office. Dense black hair shimmered in a blunt cut reaching her shoulders. A slender gold chain hung around her neck, and she wore matching gold earrings. Her makeup was subtle and tasteful, in the manner of one who is aware of her elegance but has no need to flaunt it.

"I believe my appointment was scheduled for two hours ago," she said, in English that was impeccably refined, but with an accent unplaceable to me. I offered up my rote apologies and stifled a yawn behind my palm. Ms. Houwari could have been Middle Eastern, or maybe Indian. As she spoke, I discovered why it was impossible to pin her to one locale: She had been born into a Moroccan Muslim family. She was raised in Brussels. She attended university in Paris. She was now studying for an MBA in New York City while working part-time at a Manhattan real estate company. She spoke Arabic, French, English, and Flemish.

The reason for her visit was her upcoming wedding in two months. "My fiancé would be here too," she said, folding her hands over her black leather purse, "but the bank called a sudden meeting and he wasn't able to leave the office. We wanted to do all the testing together."

As I performed the physical exam, I wondered why Nazira Houwari had come to Bellevue for medical care. She certainly appeared to have impressive financial means. Was she just taking advantage of the lower rates that Bellevue charged? Or maybe appearances were deceiving, and she was in greater financial straits than her pedigree would suggest?

In any case, she was entirely healthy, with a perfectly normal physical exam—the kind of patient that is a gift to a primary-care physician, especially one running so late. I'd be able to wrap this one up quickly and get out of clinic in time for day-care pickup.

I handed her the paper for her lab tests "Well, that's about everything," I said, pushing back my chair to get up. But then I noticed that she didn't match my movements to end the visit.

I reluctantly pulled my chair back up to my desk. "Do you have any more questions?" I asked.

"No," she said with a sigh. "I'm just tired, I suppose. Nuptial planning is rather straining."

"Are you under a lot of pressure with this wedding?" I asked.

She fingered the gold clasp on her trim leather purse. "Well, our mothers are doing most of the work, but still.... You know how it is, don't you?"

I nodded, thinking back to the flood of details that had overwhelmed Benjy and me a decade ago, when we'd planned our wedding. "Yes, it's hard to avoid the stress of that."

"Our mothers have invited a full thirty percent of the population of the EU and northern Africa. Everybody has six opinions of how it should be, and nary a soul is shy about voicing them." Ms. Houwari sank slightly in her chair. Then, seeming to think better of it, she straightened back up to her original pristine posture. "Did you have a big wedding?" she asked. Before I could answer, she added, "You're Jewish, right? Did you have a big Jewish wedding?"

"Yes," I said with a tired smile. "I am Jewish." I was too drained to think about politics. "Our wedding was big enough for me, but probably only small on the Jewish-wedding scale."

Ms. Houwari leaned forward, animated now. "So you know what it's like. It's exactly the same at a Muslim wedding—every cousin fifteen times removed needs to be invited, plus their children and their children's children's cousins. It has to be religious enough to accommodate the most conservative members of the family. Shukri and I just want a modest wedding, but it's not going to be possible." Her manicured hands moved with the rhythm of her speech. "The sum of money for this affair is outlandish. I'd rather we invest in a home, or a savings account for our future children." She spread her hands in resignation. "But our families desire a memorable event, so an event it will be."

I commiserated with her, thinking how similar "ethnic" weddings could be. I recalled Chinese and Indian friends with large, involved families, how they'd faced so many comparable challenges. Angst-laden, yes. But dull, never.

I wished Ms. Houwari luck with her wedding and directed her to the lab for her blood tests. As she walked down the hall, I could see the attention of all the passersby momentarily engaged, then slightly intimidated, by her elegant carriage and amaranthine beauty.

As soon as she was gone, I grabbed my coat and bag and then

checked the time as I tugged my door shut. Five minutes to six—I might still be able to make it. For the entire week I'd been carrying my benefits packet in my bag, and I had to get it to the department's administrator. It was due yesterday, but yesterday had been worse than today.

Most of the elevators in the old Bellevue building had been renovated by now, but the one that led to the administration area was evidently last on that list. I leaned back against worn wooden walls as the elevator ground listlessly upward, feeling the strands of the day knot around me. This was always the moment when I was assaulted by doubts. Had I remembered to review everyone's labs? Check for interactions between medications? Order the screening mammograms and colonoscopies? Had I offered HIV testing to the appropriate patients? Inquired about smoking, domestic violence, depression, and pain levels—as required for every patient?

I'd once read an editorial that calculated it would take thirty hours for an internist to cover all the required screening tests for a typical day's worth of patients. And that didn't even include discussing the diseases the patients already had. And for sure it didn't include working through interpreters and dealing with malfunctioning computers, intrusive phone calls, and piddlingly slow elevators.

I arrived at the sixth floor to see the administrator locking her office door. Mustering my most earnest smile, I scurried over and pressed the packet of papers into her hand. She flicked her eyes toward the top page—expressionless—then toward me. Finally she exhaled just deeply enough so that I knew I'd passed the test, this time at least, and unlocked her door to bring the packet inside.

I flew back down the hall hoping to catch the elevator, but unfortunately the 6:00 p.m. meridian had been crossed. The elevators were now locked, so I was left with the stairs. Some people hated the stairs, but I loved the solitude, as well as the view. The architects of 1903 believed in windows. At each turn of the stairs I was rewarded with a wide-open view of the East River and a twilight sky from which the day was fitfully draining.

The bottom of the stairs let me out at the mezzanine—a quiet wing of transomed doors and sixteen-foot ceilings. This had been one of my favorite escapes during internship. I walked now along the quiet, echoing hall toward the marble staircase that led to the ground floor, passing the three chapels. The same architects who'd graced the stairwells with such "unnecessary" accoutrements as windows had also allocated space for three wood-paneled, stained-glassed chapels. These days, only the Catholic and Protestant chapels got much use. The Jewish chapel was something of a relic, reflecting the large Jewish immigrant population in New York City when the building had been constructed, a population that had largely moved on—geographically and economically.

The great wooden doors of the chapels were closed at this hour, but the old-fashioned keyholes and the slits between the ill-fitting doors were large enough to peek through. If I squinted my eye at just the right angle, I could see the pile of untouched issues of the *Jewish Daily Forward* neatly stacked behind the last pew of the Jewish chapel.

What a strange day it had been. I couldn't recall another clinic day in which religion had come up so frequently and so openly. It dawned on me that in the religious sphere, I was a distinct minority compared with my patients. Aside from Efrain Jimenez, I could think of only two other of my patients who were Jewish, out of the many hundreds who make up my practice. Both were Russian, entirely nonreligious, and carried the aura of turn-of-the-century Lower East Side immigrants. It was only Mr. Jimenez who wished me *chag sameach* (happy holiday) on the lesser-known holidays like Tu B'shvat and Shminei Atzeret.

Bellevue now had many Muslim patients and had belatedly added a Muslim chapel at the end of this hall. Unfortunately, that chapel couldn't match the scalloped windows and arched ceilings of the other chapels that had been built into the original blueprints. It was an ordinary room converted into a modest carpeted space for prayer, but it was a popular destination for both patients and staff.

I ran my hand along the smooth marble handrail as I rounded toward the final stairwell. By demographic rights, I thought, the Jewish chapel should probably be converted to a Muslim chapel. You couldn't even make the argument anymore that the doctors were all Jewish. When I'd started at Bellevue twenty years ago, the majority of the attending physicians were Jewish. Even those who weren't, though, mostly hailed from the Upper West Side and knew their Nova from their belly lox and their *schlemiels* from their *schlimazels*. Now, probably only about a third of the faculty in our clinic was Jewish; this was directly related to the demographics of the residency program, which had shifted over the years to Asian and Southeast Asian. Maybe only 10 percent of the house staff was Jewish these days.

I trotted down the wide marble steps that were smoothed concave from a century of footfalls. What, then, did it mean to be a minority? To some degree, everyone at Bellevue was a minority—whether religious or ethnic—within larger American society: Muslims, Jews, Hindus, Catholics, Buddhists, blacks, Hispanics, Asians. Patients didn't blink when their doctors had odd, unpronounceable names. Interns didn't see much unusual when their patients spoke languages they'd never heard of. Hospital chaplains could perform rituals in almost any faith. In fact, the only numerical minority at Bellevue was probably the white Anglo-Saxon Protestant; there were hardly any patients, doctors, or administrators who fit that bill.

I left the hospital and started toward day care, stopping at the fruit cart to pick up bananas for tomorrow's lunches. Jamil—the regular guy—had gone back to Pakistan for two months, as he did every year. Each year upon his return he'd announce that a new baby was on the way. But he could never be there for the birth.

I didn't know the fellow who was running the stand in his absence—maybe it was a friend or a cousin. He was nice enough, but it just wasn't the same. Jamil had become a part of my children's lives because of his strategic location between home and day care. That meant that twice a day, every day, there was a free banana or stick of gum. Jamil made sure he stocked the sugarless type in the special spot under the stand so that my kids could root it out.

In so many aspects of our culture, it seemed, we were driven by finding the commonality of religion or ethnicity. But at Bellevue, this factionalizing didn't seem to be the case. Maybe it was because there wasn't any single dominant group; everyone was a little bit out of the mainstream in one manner or another. I imagined that this easygoing chaos probably seemed startling to immigrants arriving from societies in which racial, ethnic, and social distinctions were marginalizing, threatening, or even murderous.

I purchased my bananas and jogged the last few blocks to day care. I didn't want to be late yet again.

The next morning was so rushed that it wasn't until I'd arrived at the hospital that I realized I'd forgotten to eat breakfast. In the buzz of feeding Naava, Noah, Ariel, and Juliet, I'd somehow neglected to feed myself, and now I was starving. I rummaged in my drawer and found a package of dried mangoes that one of my patients had brought back from her visit home to the Philippines. This would suffice; then I could easily fast until lunchtime. My pathetic fast brought to mind Mr. Jimenez and Mr. Sarkhel, both citing their respective fasting holidays to reassure me that they'd lose the weight they needed to. I wondered if Ramadan and Yom Kippur actually offered any net health benefits to the city of New York. I could envision the Department of Health working on this. Would Lent count? What about the nineteen-day Baha'i fast? What about the fasts in Jainism and Hinduism?

Then suddenly it hit me. Yom Kippur was next week. A foreboding feeling crept over me: had I canceled my patients for that day? Every year I always blocked off that day well in advance, but I couldn't remember doing it this year. I quickly checked my schedule and there it was—a full panel of patients. Damn!

The clinic required that we give a minimum of ninety days' notice before canceling any session, but in all the chaos of returning from Costa Rica and settling into New York life with three kids instead of two, the whole thing had slipped my mind, and now the holiday was next week. What an idiot I was!

I scanned the list of patients. Half did not speak English. At least three did not have phone numbers listed. I knew that many did not have answering machines. Four were patients I'd never met before.

The truth was, I was not a religious person, so it was hard to argue that this day off was a religious necessity. It wouldn't be fair to inconvenience all my patients, even potentially putting their health at risk. Nor could I simply call in sick on short notice and saddle my non-Jewish colleagues with my patients.

Still, this was Yom Kippur. Even the most assimilated Jew in the world knew that this was the holiest day of the Jewish calendar. I'd always stayed home from work or school on Yom Kippur, even if I didn't go to synagogue. Intellectually I was well aware of the contradiction, yet it was just what I did. It was Yom Kippur. Period.

But I had to admit that this was ridiculous. I wasn't religious. I wasn't going to spend the day in synagogue. I probably wouldn't even fast—well, maybe until lunchtime. How could I make the argument that I needed this day off if I was just going to stay home and read the *New York Times*?

It was an obvious conclusion that my obligation to my patients overrode any religious obligation. Plus the Torah had all sorts of dispensations when it came to doctoring. I could surely justify this. That Wednesday I did something I'd never done in my entire life—I went to work on Yom Kippur.

The clinic was quiet, with many rooms darkened. I felt like I was walking on spongy, sodden ground. I chided myself for feeling awkward. It was just a regular day, I told myself. I pulled out my first batch of charts and when I turned the corner toward my office, I ran smack into Sarah, another physician. We both jumped, as though we'd been caught hoarding slabs of bacon dripping with melted cheese. We smiled nervously at each other, and then she said, "You too?"

We crept off to our respective offices with the unspoken need to keep a low profile. I tried to behave as though it were a normal day, but my patients did not permit this.

"Aren't you supposed to be home today?" Mr. Villanueva asked.

"Shouldn't you be fasting?" asked Ms. Deng.

"How come you aren't at synagogue?" Mrs. Escobar asked.

"Isn't this the holiest day of the year?" Mr. Dumbaya asked.

When it comes to Yom Kippur, it seemed, everybody was a Jewish grandmother.

Sheepishly, I explained my scheduling error. I gave the whole megillah about forgetting to block the session, the required ninety-day advance notice, the inability to contact everyone at the last minute, my reasoning regarding my priorities, and so forth. All the patients said that they would have understood if they'd shown up and I wasn't there.

"It's more important," Mr. Alhadji insisted, "that you do the right thing for your religion than show up for work."

"You have to pay attention to your people and your history," said Mr. Lutysaski.

"You have to set an example for your children," Mrs. Perez said.

"What would Moses do?" said Leonard Daniels, a slouching college student wearing a backward Malcolm X baseball hat.

I thanked one and all for their concerns and their generosity of spirit but endeavored to focus on their medical issues rather than my religious lapses.

Perliana Josephs was my last patient of the day. "Don't mess yourself up next year, Dr. Ofri," she said. "God's watching. You know that, right?"

The very next day I blocked off Yom Kippur for next year—364 days in advance—just to be on the safe side. I couldn't verify whether or not God was watching, but I knew for sure that my patients were.

∽ Chapter Eighteen ∽

Despite my best intentions of keeping an open mind, on the following Monday afternoon, when I read that my next patient was Mohammed Ali Amal, I couldn't suppress my mental image of the iconic American boxer. The man who answered to this name, however, bore no resemblance to him in any way. Gaunt and rawboned, he had a concave torso that seemed too slight to tether his four lanky limbs. A dense thicket of eyebrows shadowed his recessed black eyes and haggard face, which was covered with a dark swath of stubble. His angular nose was prominent, and its sharp deviation to the right did not seem natural. He was only thirty-seven, but his steps were the cautious steps of an older man, and he seemed to consider carefully before sitting in the seat I offered him in my office. When he sat down, he folded his arms and legs into himself, hunching his shoulders into his scooped-out chest, minimizing the cubic footage he occupied.

When I asked where he was from, his voice came out in a whisper. "Iraq."

Mr. Amal had grown up in a relatively secular family in Baghdad. He'd studied computer science at the university and worked at various times for the United Nations and the World Health Organization doing information technology. He had several clients in Jordan and had spent most of the war living and working there.

A year ago, he'd decided to go back to Iraq for a week to visit his family. His friends warned him not to go, that it was dangerous, but he hadn't seen his family in years and it would only be for a week.

"They came looking for me," he said in a cramped, scratchy voice that was bereft of color and intonation. "They came to an office where I was visiting friends, specifically looking for me. My friends said I wasn't there, but they hunted the building until they found me hiding behind boxes in a closet." His voice barely rustled the air around him.

He couldn't really tell me who "they" were, but his crime was obvious: working for an organization that had connections to the Americans. For twenty-one days he was held in a cellar and beaten. Nobody interrogated him for information; they simply beat him daily on his feet, on his face, on his legs, on his back. They used metal poles, wooden sticks, wires, and fists.

I tried to keep the images at bay, but all I could see was Mr. Amal's slight body lost in a sea of "them"—the pounding of bats and fists, the dull give of muscle and bone, screams muted, blood smeared. Knowing that there were hundreds, thousands, of similar situations occurring with banality all over Iraq, all over the world, was one thing. But to look at a specific person and envision that human being within that melee of brutality was another thing altogether. I felt cowardly that Costa Rica came to me at that moment. Yes, all the cruelty of the world would still be occurring even if I spinelessly retreated to the red-tiled veranda and ensconced myself under the cascades of bougainvillea. But that didn't stop me from wishing.

Friends and colleagues from the WHO collected money for a ransom, and Mr. Amal was finally released, barely able to walk. He returned to Jordan as soon as he could physically mobilize himself. Three months later he came to the United States with the help of an American acquaintance who lived in a small town near Newark, New Jersey.

There are so many metaphors for how people appear after a traumatic event—being shadows of their former selves, or having a hollowness in their souls. These are only metaphors, but they seemed physically accurate descriptions of Mr. Amal. He actually looked like a shadow—so fragilely constructed that he might crumple in the wind. His carriage did indeed seem hollow, as though I could pass a hand through him, through a void of body and soul. Something had been eviscerated from him by those torturers.

Mr. Amal started out living with his friend, then eventually got his own apartment nearby. But there were no Iraqis, no Arabs of any sort, in that random New Jersey suburb. He found himself completely isolated and lonely, utterly baffled by American culture.

"Nobody talks to you in America," he said, kneading the tips of his bony fingers. "They are polite and greet you—'Hi, how are you?'—but they don't actually want an answer. Nobody ever has a conversation. Nobody invites you to their home. In Baghdad, no matter how horrible things were—with Saddam Hussein, with the war—people always invited you to their homes to share a meal. I've never seen the inside of a single home in America. Not one." His fingers finally settled in his lap, limp with disappointment.

To earn money, Mr. Amal tried to continue his IT work with clients in Jordan. In order to coordinate the time difference he had to stay up most of the night. He'd then sleep most of the day, further isolating himself from the world. His only real contacts were the phone conversations he had with family in Iraq. "Cell phones are the only things left in the entire country that work," he said with a bitter smile.

Mr. Amal had seen the psychiatrist as part of the SOT program but, like Azad Aptekin, wasn't comfortable with the idea of needing help or taking medications. He had no other medical conditions and had always been in excellent health up until the "accident," as he referred to it. The only specific thing that was bothering him now was restless legs when he tried to sleep in the mornings.

I contemplated this shadow of a man—a shadow trailed by its own bitter shadow of his sufferings. How could I help this man? I wasn't a psychiatrist, and even if I were, how was it possible to undo such pain?

I gave him a prescription for gabapentin, the one medication we stocked in the Bellevue pharmacy that might help restless legs and nerve-type pain. Mr. Amal gave a formal bow before he shuffled out the door. The thin paper prescription grasped in his right hand seemed symbolic of the inadequacy of humanity. Was that all we could offer him—just a few pills?

Viseltear Violins was located on the corner of Essex and Rivington, a section of the Lower East Side that was a decided mix of the hoary and the hip. The Streit's Matzo factory, a Chinese herbalist, and a bulk-candy vendor shared these blocks with urbane bistros and European couture shops. The violin workshop sat above an all-purpose pharmacy and small-appliance store whose window was lined with dusty blenders and assorted stomach remedies. I hauled my cello three flights up a wide wooden staircase, each step heaving with tectonic magnitude. The staircase was easily more than a century old, but when I creaked open the door to the workshop, I felt as though I'd been transported even several centuries earlier.

Late-afternoon sun crept through unadorned casement windows onto ancient, sawdust-strewn floorboards. Bodies of cellos, violas, and violins in various stages of construction hung placidly from rods running along the ceiling. Curved wooden molds were fastened to the walls. Rutted workbenches lined the perimeter of the small workshop. Instrument body parts stuck out from vises, calipers, and clamps at various angles. Tins of glues, varnishes, lacquers, and stains, syruplike dribbles solidified to the sides, formed a haphazard skyline in one corner. An old-fashioned hutch with a hundred little drawers overflowed with pegs, tuners, bridges, screws of all sizes and shapes. Thick planks of spruce and maple teetered in stacks. Bows of all lengths dangled from racks. Saws, files, reamers, shavers were strewn about, with a sense of being caught in mid-action.

Sebastian, the luthier, examined my cello with the care and sureness of a neonatologist handling a preemie. He was a lanky fellow, with a meditative, almost monkish air about him. I'd expected an elderly man, someone descended from an esteemed family of luthiers, a vestigial artisan who could exist in our modern world only as a quaint holdover from an earlier era in Vienna, perhaps, or Cremona. But Sebastian was in his midthirties and wore jeans and Converse high-tops underneath his stained calf-length apron. He'd studied art restoration in his native Romania but shifted to violin making a decade ago after he'd had a happenstance exposure to the luthier trade upon immigrating to America. He had a natural finesse, an instinct for stringed instruments, though he himself did not play.

For the past few months I'd noticed a buzz in my cello strings. It occurred only at certain moments, but it was like a car alarm discombobulating my concentration. I was sure that it was a loose peg or a wobbly tailpiece, but I'd tightened every part of the cello that could be tightened with no discernible improvement. The buzz didn't occur all the time, so I sometimes wondered if I was a musical hypochondriac. I finally decided to approach the problem methodically, checking each note on the instrument. The buzz indeed occurred only occasionally, but there turned out to be a method to the madness: it only arose when I played an E. Interestingly, the same buzzing occurred whether I played an E on the D string or an E on the G string.

"It's not a mechanical issue of the strings," Sebastian said when I related this odd finding. "Something in the architecture of your cello is reacting to the particular resonance of an E." He lifted the cello onto a workbench. I was grateful that someone was able to reassure me that I wasn't hallucinating.

Sebastian squatted to be at eye level with the instrument, squinting as he ran a finger up and down the ebony neck. He nodded to himself, and then straightened up. He loosened the pegs of my cello and within seconds had peeled back all the strings. The cello looked naked and I couldn't suppress my twinge of empathy for it. Sebastian pulled a metal ruler out from a pocket in his apron and rested it along the plane of the now bare fingerboard. He rotated the ruler, measuring angles with just his eye. He turned the cello on its side, inspecting and palpating the body. I remained silent, loath to interrupt a master diagnostician at work. Sebastian reminded me of some of the older attendings from the "days of the giants" who could diagnose any patient with a precise physical exam—no wimpy MRIs or echocardiograms.

"There's a warp in the topography of the fingerboard," Sebastian concluded. He motioned me to crouch down and match his visual perspective on the neck of the cello, but I was not able to perceive the subtle distortion that he saw. "The warp has a specific physical quality that creates a buzz when there is a vibration frequency of E or any of its multiples."

Sebastian spent the next hour sanding, molding, measuring, and adjusting my cello, treating it as though it were a Stradivarius rather than the midlevel student cello that it was. With a feather-thin paintbrush he touched up minor flaws in the lacquer that were invisible to my eye. He polished with three different grades of cloth.

As I sat silently watching my cello being restored to health, I thought about Mohammed Ali Amal. It seemed supremely unfair that a hollow piece of wood could merit such gentle and respectful treatment while human beings could be treated as refuse. How could someone take his body—perfectly healthy, cared for, and loved—and smash it to pieces?

Sebastian reattached the strings, tuned them, and then gently placed the cello in my arms—I was again reminded of the neonatologist. "Try it," he said, and I took up the bow. The strings sounded rich and melodious. The buzz was vastly diminished, but unfortunately still present. Sebastian shook his head, his disappointment patent and profound. "No," he said, "it's not good enough."

He took the cello from me and again laid it on the bench. He gazed at it without speaking for five solid minutes. Then he rested his hand against the curved scroll. "The pegs may need to be refitted, but I'm not sure. I might file down the bridge, see if we can smooth the angle a bit. And the endpin seems like it's under a lot of tension from the tailpiece. I could adjust it, or maybe there's an extra tailpiece lying around here and I could just replace it. Do you mind leaving the cello overnight?"

The hesitation must have been obvious on my face.

"Don't worry," Sebastian said. "I will take good care of it."

I was sure that he would, and I climbed down the creaky tenement steps knowing that my child was in safe hands. It was a confidence that sat warmly in my chest, a confidence I knew that I was lucky to have.

∾ Chapter Nineteen ∾

"Mr. Ptchet...," I called. I glanced at the clock while I tried to figure out how to pronounce *Ptchetpchdad*. Three patients still to go and day-care pickup time was in less than an hour. "Ptchet...pchdad?" I knew I was mispronouncing good portions of the name and I couldn't even hazard a guess as to what ethnicity I'd be looking for. Eastern European? North African? Scandinavian? Caribbean? Baltic?

"Ptchetpchdad?" I said again, recasting my syllabic emphasis, hoping I might land on a closer approximation of the name. Heads and necks craned toward me, faces screwed, straining to match my mangled utterances to their own names.

Finally a stout man rose from the crowd. He had a full fleshy face, his pitch-black skin pockmarked from acne. He wore a beige trench coat over faded dress pants and sneakers.

I pointed to the printed name on the chart to be sure it was him—I'd already suffered the misfortune of trusting my pronunciation and ending up with the wrong patient in my room—and then started walking toward my office. He didn't follow but instead reached into his nylon athletic bag and hunted until he retrieved a blue passport—République du Cameroun. I nodded in acknowledgment, hoping to hurry him along, but he flipped painstakingly through the pages until he found his photo and pressed the passport to me. Thierry Ptchetpchdad stared out somberly in black-and-white, with his name handwritten underneath in elaborate script.

I handed back the passport and briskly led Mr. Ptchetpchdad back to my office, hoping he was in possession of a good walking pace, a reasonable slice of the English language, and general good health.

I apologized to him for the delay and then steeled myself for efficiency. *I'll resist all small talk,* I swore to myself. *Cut him off at the pass if he starts to ramble.*

As Mr. Ptchetpchdad settled himself after hanging up his coat and stowing his athletic bag, I quickly scanned the computerized medical record. He was a sixty-year-old man who appeared to come to clinic once a year, each time seeing a different doctor. I could see that his medical history included hepatitis C and a renal cyst, but he wasn't on any medications. A small flame of cheer flickered inside me as I calculated that I'd be able to shave a few minutes off the visit by not having to write any prescriptions.

"English?" I asked hopefully, and he shook his head.

"Español?" I tried, remembering Aristide Mezondes, who'd learned Spanish in the Congo. Mr. Ptchetpchdad stared at me blankly.

"Français?" He nodded, and I was already dialing extension 1800 and pressing #2, hoping to get connected to Evans. But luck wasn't with me today. Through the interpreter, I asked the gentleman from Cameroon what he was here for.

"To get everything checked" was the answer. "I want to know about all cancers, and cholesterol and everything I need."

"Okay," I said, calculating how long it might take to cover "everything." "Let's briefly review your medical history. I see here that you have hepatitis C. Have you ever had treatment for that?"

"What is that, Doctor?" came the reply. "I do not understand."

"Hepatitis," I repeated. "Hepatitis C."

"What is hepatitis, Doctor?"

"It's an infection of the liver," I said. "Were you ever told of an infection of the liver?"

"No, Doctor. I never had any infection of the liver."

Shit, I said to myself as the solid ground of a straightforward medical visit began to crumble. Was the patient wrong, or was the medical record wrong? I hurriedly scrolled through the past laboratory values while the patient and the interpreter waited on the line. I uncovered several confirmatory antibody tests over the past seven years and breathed a small sigh of relief that at least we doctors hadn't made a bald error. "Are you sure?" I asked, trying to speak more gently. "You've had quite a number of blood tests showing that you've had hepatitis."

"I have never had any liver infection," Mr. Ptchetpchdad insisted.

I started from the beginning, explaining about the liver, and the several types of hepatitis, and the blood tests. Each phrase went back and forth via the interpreter as the clock ticked relentlessly forward. During the linguistic loop-the-loops, I scoured the computer for more lab data.

Someone had checked his viral load, and it turned out that there was no actual virus left in his blood, just the antibody. So maybe his body had cleared the infection years ago and he'd simply forgotten about the diagnosis. I could feel my mind clearing as something about his behavior and the clinical picture appeared to make sense.

Most of our twenty minutes had elapsed and I hadn't even completed the review of his past medical history, let alone addressed his current concerns. Not to mention the physical exam. Plus the two other patients waiting.

I excused myself and stepped into the hallway to call day care and let them know I'd be late. I left a message for my husband, hoping he could make the day-care pickup for Noah and Ariel in addition to getting Naava at her elementary school, which was in the complete opposite direction. The circuitous route with three hungry, tired, cranky children at the end of the day could take an hour, the type of hour that made airport security lines seem like a pleasant diversion.

I returned to my office and picked up the phone with the interpreter to plow through the rest of Mr. Ptchetpchdad's medical history as quickly as I could. Mr. Ptchetpchdad nodded when I read off the parts about glaucoma and back pain, but when I mentioned the kidney cyst that was listed in the previous note, he looked at me blankly.

Not again. *Doesn't he know anything that's ever happened to his body? Did someone pay this guy to make my life miserable?* Trying to keep my voice steady through gritted teeth, I reviewed the numerous ultrasounds he'd had over the years that showed a cyst. I felt a little guilty, because a simple renal cyst was probably an incidental finding, so maybe that was why he didn't remember. But still!

Mr. Ptchetpchdad was otherwise healthy—at least something in my favor. I started on his request for colon cancer screening.

Usually, when I explained what a colonoscopy was, I wriggled my pinky to indicate both the diameter of the scope and the approximate direction that it traveled. Some things were difficult to convey via a telephone interpreter.

But somehow Mr. Ptchetpchdad seemed to catch on right away and enthusiastically said that he would want the colonoscopy. I was typing faster now, skipping ahead to the physical exam fields even though we hadn't done the exam yet. I'd hazard a guess that his exam would be largely normal, and could always go back later and fix anything that wasn't.

I debated about whether to embark on the issue of prostate cancer screening. The correct conversation about prostate cancer screening was a prolonged and sophisticated discussion about the high false-positive and false-negative rates. To achieve true informed consent, I had to discuss prostate cancer itself, how some cancers were so slow growing that they didn't need to be treated and others were aggressive, but the test couldn't distinguish between these. That treatment for prostate cancer had significant side effects (incontinence and impotence) that might outweigh the benefits. That if Mr. Ptchetpchdad was the type of person who would never want a treatment with those side effects, then he shouldn't do the PSA test, but if he was a person who would want aggressive treatment no matter what the risks, then he should do the test, although he should understand that even a negative test result wouldn't completely rule out cancer.

Day care charged a dollar a minute when you were late—which wasn't nearly as bad as the forlorn look on your kids' faces as they sat by the door, the last ones remaining, while the janitors were sweeping, the lights were being dimmed, and the last teacher was nervously fingering her keys.

I was immediately ambushed by guilt. Clinically, the PSA discussion was the exact right thing to do. Mr. Ptchetpchdad was an appropriate candidate for screening—he was relatively young and healthy, and Africans, in fact, had a slightly higher risk of prostate cancer. *Do the right thing,* I told myself, shoveling down my aching desire to finish up quickly and pick up my children.

I plunged into the PSA conversation and immediately regretted it. The La Brea tar pits would have been easier to wade through. Mr. Ptchetpchdad kept saying yes to everything I said, but it was obvious that he didn't have a clue. After garbling around with him for what felt like an hour, I finally took his yes at face value and ordered the PSA in the computer along with the cholesterol he'd requested.

Then I started the colonoscopy-ordering process—two excruciating pages of fine print to be filled out by hand—keeping my muttered curses at subaudible level. Our colonoscopists were the last Luddites of Bellevue, refusing to accept computerized requests. Printing the patient's first name, last name, medical record number, medications—things that were all in the computer—always put me in a foul mood, especially when I was running late. "Do the right thing," I kept snarling under my breath to keep from tossing the whole damn thing in the garbage.

Forty-five minutes had now elapsed, but at least I could take mild comfort in the fact that I had done a thorough job. Before I hung up the phone with the translator, I asked the patient if he had any further questions. The interpreter relayed the answer: "I would like to thank you for the superior medical care I am receiving here. You are a most excellent medical doctor and I thank you ever so much."

My fingers slid off the computer keys and I immediately flushed with embarrassment. Here I was cursing throughout this entire encounter, and Mr. Ptchetpchdad was appreciative and gracious. I had really sunk low.

Needless to say, I was more than relieved to rise from my chair and escort Mr. Ptchetpchdad at a sprinter's pace out to the clerk who would take care of his appointments. Back in my office, I took a few deep breaths, appreciating the minute of solitude before the next patient was called in. I still had to finish the assessment and plan sections in Mr. Ptchetpchdad's note before I could get to the next patient, so I gathered the last remnants of my focus and tried to power through as fast as I could.

As I was typing, it hit me that I'd completely forgotten to do the physical exam. I slammed both fists on the desk in unison, and my plastic specimen cup full of paper clips clattered to the floor.

I scrolled back to the physical exam section on the computer and jabbed the delete button on everything I'd painstakingly entered. All I had were the vital signs taken by the medical assistant: *BP 138/85, height 5'6", weight 173 lbs.* That would have to do; there was no way I was going to call that man back into my room.

An inadvertent click brought me to an earlier progress note from two years before, and I saw a reference to a discussion about screening for cholesterol. And then another about PSA testing. And then another about colonoscopy—the exact same discussions I'd just painfully navigated with him while my children were being hauled out of the day-care building and plopped on the sidewalk along with the sacks of trash.

Jolted by a wave of fury, I started actively hunting down test results in our frustratingly disjointed electronic medical record system. Searching for PSA, I discovered a normal result from last year. Searching for the cholesterol uncovered normal results from two years ago. Then I started looking into the colonoscopy—a test that was generally needed every ten years. There it was: two years ago. Perfectly normal colonoscopy.

It was one thing to forget about blood tests for PSA and cholesterol, even hepatitis. But no one forgets having a three-foot tube threaded up his or her rectum. How could Mr. Ptchetpchdad have watched me painstakingly fill out the colonoscopy forms by hand and not once pipe up and say, "Oh yes, I've had one of those before," as any other patient would?

I shoved the forms in the garbage, then swung a swift kick at the pail for good measure. Do the right thing, indeed! My kids were probably wandering along Twenty-third Street shaking tin cups at passersby. I was furious at both him and myself.

I fumed through my last two patients. I fumed as I stormed out of the hospital in the darkness, arriving home as my children—evidently rescued from the gutter—were being tucked into bed. I fumed as I read through *Runaway Bunny*. Let the goddamn rabbit make it on his own.

It was only when I settled into my own bed, late that night, that the tension began to ease. There is something about being horizontal that allows the mind to unclench. I'm convinced there's some sort of neuronal upset once the cranium is knocked flat on its back, a salutary spillage of neurotransmitters leaching out of the synapses, draining into the netherworld of a goose-down pillow.

I wondered if perhaps I'd been overreacting with Mr. Ptchetpchdad just a mite. Maybe he had a cognitive impairment that caused him not to remember his colonoscopy and his hepatitis and his renal cyst and his PSA and his cholesterol. It certainly would be rather cruel of me—a physician—to be angry if there was a biological basis to his forgetfulness.

Or maybe he was an utter idiot, demanding whatever test he wanted, regardless of the cost in dollars—which he'd never pay—or the cost in my time.

—⊗⊗⊗—

The next day I was still annoyed. I starting telling the experience to one of my colleagues in the clinic, but the story was so convoluted and took so much effort to get across that I gave up after the renal cyst. It was just going to have to be one of those things that took place in the privacy of a doctor's office. Nobody would ever know or care about all the effort I'd put in to do the right thing, or that I'd missed picking up my kids, or that I'd harbored evil thoughts about the runaway bunny. I'd just have to chalk this one up and move on.

Then it dawned on me that there had indeed been someone who shared that experience with me, that I hadn't been truly alone in my misery: the interpreter had been there with me.

Now that I'd made contact with Evans, I no longer thought of the interpreters as faceless entities, evanescent beings who evaporated once the phone was restored to its cradle. I dialed the interpreter service and pressed #2 for French. When I described my patient encounter to the interpreter who answered, she asked around and eventually my interpreter was located.

"I just need to resolve one thing," I said. "Did that gentleman from Cameroon have any sort of cognitive impairment that you could tell?"

"Well, he seemed sort of simple," the interpreter replied. "I don't think he had any mental problems, if that's what you are wondering, but he kept asking the same things over and over again."

I proceeded to unload my pent-up frustration about the hepatitis and the renal cyst and the PSA and the colonoscopy. The interpreter was patient with me, offering murmurs of understanding as I described how much effort I'd put in and how it felt all wasted due to Mr. Ptchetpchdad's seeming lack of awareness and how it made everything run late and how I couldn't get out in time to pick up my kids and how I'd missed dinner with them. On and on I went, feeling my anger gradually dissipate as I poured out my woes to this remarkably tolerant stranger at the other end of the line.

At the end of the conversation, I concluded that Mr. Ptchetpchdad was a bit simpleminded, maybe a bit self-involved, maybe a bit confused about all that was going on—but that he was just one point on the bell curve of personalities, whether he came from Cameroon, Copenhagen, or Connecticut. I was somewhere on that same bell curve, with my own amalgam of personality traits, and we just didn't have a smooth synergy between us.

"But," the interpreter commented, "he was very, very appreciative of his medical care. He repeated that several times."

I sighed and hung up the phone. I'd just have to be satisfied that at least one thing had gone well with Mr. Ptchetpchdad.

Chapter Twenty

Intern shorthand would describe Juan Moreno as a sixty-seven-year-old male with MMP—multiple medical problems. He had the trifecta of diabetes, hypertension, and elevated cholesterol, topped with cardiomyopathy, atrial fibrillation, obesity, arthritis, sleep apnea, and asthma. His heart pumped at only a third of the normal capacity and, like Julia Barquero's, required a panoply of medications to keep episodes of congestive heart failure at bay.

When Mr. Moreno first had a heart attack and atrial fibrillation, at age fifty-three, he was discharged from Bellevue with the standard appointment slip: *Medical Clinic with any MD*. By the random luck of the draw, that "any MD" turned out to be me, an intern fresh out of medical school.

Mr. Moreno was unfailingly cheerful at his appointments, a reliable burst of sunshine no matter how chaotic or miserable the day. Though he was fully comfortable speaking English with me, Mr. Moreno's English retained the inflection, sentence structure, and rhythm of Puerto Rican Spanish.

Many of my patients drifted in and out over the years. Some had socioeconomic barriers to maintaining consistent care. Some moved back to their native countries. Some were homeless or nearly so. Some had lives disjointed by alcohol, depression, divorce, or financial calamity.

But not Mr. Moreno. He'd lived with his wife of fifty years in the same public-housing apartment for all the time I'd known him. He'd worked for twenty-seven years at the same factory. He'd maintained the same phone number, the same address, the same schedule, the same commute. His phone always worked. Messages always got answered. Prescriptions always got filled. Referrals and follow-up appointments were always carried out. In his entirely unprepossessing and self-deprecating manner, he was the epitome of reliable. My longest-term doctor-patient relationship was with Juan Moreno.

Despite his MMP, Mr. Moreno was functioning remarkably well. He was able to do most of the things he wanted. He made it back to Puerto Rico whenever possible to visit family. He relished summer visits to the Poconos. He loved raucous family picnics by the East River with mountains of food and relatives, and a radio blaring Latin Top 40.

But there was always a risk of something bad happening. People with MMP lived a fragile truce with illness—at any moment one pillar in the tower could give out, and I feared for Mr. Moreno. At one of our visits I'd even raised the issues of advance directives and DNR...just in case.

One of the gravest risks of a poorly pumping heart is life-threatening arrhythmia. Ventricular tachycardia and ventricular fibrillation could lead to sudden death—unless someone happened to be standing nearby with a defibrillator in hand. That rarely being the case, cardiologists implanted defibrillators that could deliver the necessary shock from inside the body. The AICD (automatic implantable cardioverter defibrillator) monitored the heart rhythm at all times, and if a serious arrhythmia occurred, it delivered a jolt akin to an elephant stomping on the chest.

The cardiologists had been trying to convince Mr. Moreno to agree to an AICD. Mr. Moreno was leery of having anything placed inside him and sought my advice. Actually, he sought more than my advice; he wanted me to make the decision for him.

"You tell me what to do and I do it," he said flatly. "You my head doctor and I do what you say."

My reaction was to squirm at the paternalistic ramifications of what he was saying. But by now I'd become accustomed to this attitude that was so prevalent in my patients from other countries and so rare in my patients born and raised in the United States. Mr. Ptchetpchdad represented one extreme of the immigrant population, just saying yes to whatever I said, irrespective of whether he understood. But most of my immigrant patients, like Julia Barquero and Dr. Chan, were quite content to leave decision-making to me, rarely questioning my choice of medications or tests. Americans, by contrast, almost reflexively offered their opinions—positive or negative—on any medical recommendation.

With Mr. Moreno, however, the problem wasn't just my general discomfort about making a major decision for him; it was that I had real concerns as to whether an AICD was the right treatment. For one thing, we were talking about a *prophylactic* procedure, doing an intervention for a condition (a lethal cardiac arrhythmia) that had not yet occurred and for all we knew might never occur. Plus, this was an invasive procedure with small but definite risks. Why rock the boat when things were going so well right now?

If I could see into the future and know that Mr. Moreno was destined to be struck by a grave arrhythmia and suffer a sudden cardiac death, well then, this AICD would be lifesaving and I'd recommend it immediately. But the truth was that these arrhythmias only happened to a minority of patients, not all. Those unlucky patients would truly benefit from AICDs; everyone else would not. But all who got them would have to face the risks that came with the procedure.

I had no way of knowing whether the fates intended Mr. Moreno to fall into the unlucky group or the lucky group. The scientific literature could tell me what happened, on average, to a population of patients, but it couldn't tell me anything about Juan Angel Moreno, the rotund, balding, brown-eyed sixty-seven-year-old Puerto Rican man leaning forward on the wooden cane that he carried more for show than use.

My honest opinion was that the AICD could possibly help him, but I wanted to elicit Mr. Moreno's own feelings. I wanted to understand what *he* felt about the potential risks versus the potential benefits, but he seemed loath to take a stand. He wanted me to make the decision.

I pressed him about his general philosophy of life. Mr. Moreno described to me what I might call a modified fatalistic viewpoint. He was raised Catholic, and though he wasn't practicing now, his religion influenced his outlook. "What will be, will be," he told me several times. "Whatever God decides is what will happen."

But he was still willing to participate in other medical treatments that, by definition, were intended to alter his destiny. He took Coumadin to avoid blood clots from his atrial fibrillation. He took diabetes pills to lower the risks of blindness and kidney failure from high sugar levels. He took blood-pressure pills to lessen his risk of stroke. He submitted to a colonoscopy every ten years to avoid colon cancer.

But in his mind, this metal box that was to be surgically implanted into his body was in a different category, and he would do it only if I said so. I saw that I was not going to be able to coax a decision from him, so I had to try to weigh the various factors using what I understood of his values.

Mr. Moreno clearly seemed willing to take on some risks in order to obtain benefits. He had had several cardiac catheterizations in the past, so he certainly was capable of incorporating invasive procedures into his frame of reference.

He also had a lot to live for. He had a stable marriage of half a century. He had children and grandchildren in whose lives he was involved and invested. In particular, there was Cynthia. Cynthia was the adored granddaughter he'd been raising in his home since she was two. Whenever I asked about Cynthia's mother—Mr. Moreno's daughter—he'd just shake his head with monumental sadness and say, "She's on the street." Sometimes Cynthia ran into her mother in the neighborhood, and her mother wouldn't talk to her. It wasn't clear that her mother even recognized her anymore, so utterly had heroin eviscerated her life. Cynthia's father, though in prison, sent letters and kept up with monthly phone calls.

I decided that the weight of the evidence—both medical and social—suggested that the AICD was worthwhile and that overall it would offer Mr. Moreno more benefit than harm. And so I told him that I thought he should do it.

"Fine," he said. Without missing a beat, Mr. Moreno rose up from his chair, pressing slightly on the cane for assistance. "You my head doctor and I trust you. I do whatever you tell me." He left my office and walked directly to the cardiology clinic to schedule the procedure.

∽ Chapter Twenty-one ∽

Three weeks later I saw Mr. Ptchetpchdad's name on my list of appointments for the day and I cursed out loud. The clerk flashed a puzzled look at me, as I wasn't one who normally voiced expletives. I spied Mr. Ptchetpchdad in the waiting room, and my annoyance and frustration from our first visit came steaming back. What was he doing back so soon? He didn't have diabetes or hypertension or heart disease or any other chronic illness that required frequent visits. He was healthy, damn it. Didn't he appreciate that? An annual visit was more than enough for a neurotic simpleton in excellent health.

Mr. Ptchetpchdad caught my glance and began rising from his chair. His eagerness to get to my office irritated me even more. Was this going to be another forty-five-minute torture session haggling via an interpreter over multiple tests he didn't need? I could just see it now: Mr. Ptchetpchdad wondering if maybe his magnesium level was low. Mr. Ptchetpchdad requesting hair implants. Mr. Ptchetpchdad insisting on kidney surgery for his (benign) renal cyst. Mr. Ptchetpchdad interested in an MRI to make sure his pancreas was healthy. Mr. Ptchetpchdad inquiring about a liver transplant because of his (inactive) hepatitis C. Mr. Ptchetpchdad upset because the clinic pharmacy did not offer discounted Viagra. Mr. Ptchetpchdad demanding a mammogram because he'd heard that some men got breast cancer. Mr. Ptchetpchdad wondering if liposuction was available for the American-style gut he'd acquired since immigrating.

My blood pressure was rising just contemplating the session with him. I signaled Mr. Ptchetpchdad to sit back down, raising two fingers to indicate that I had two patients ahead of him.

First was a quick visit with Julia Barquero. She was here only for a blood test, but she wanted to update me on Vasco. In the end, she'd been too scared to travel to Texas because she didn't know how long the process would take. It seemed that she'd made the right decision, because her brother, who'd gone in her place, had been there for two months now.

He filed papers, paid fees, and attended hearings. He scraped money together for a lawyer. Meanwhile eight-year-old Vasco—with limited cognitive skills and no English—remained in the detention center. But because Julia's brother had a green card, he was able to sign as an official sponsor for the boy. Things looked promising, Julia said, and maybe Vasco would be able to come to New York.

I could only imagine the reaction of the nativists—another illegal immigrant rewarded for successfully breaking the law. But I was delighted.

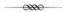

After I'd finished with the next patient—a young Sri Lankan with gastritis—Mr. Ptchetpchdad trundled into my office. He painstakingly smoothed his trench coat and hung it up on the hook. He rifled through his athletic bag while I tapped my foot impatiently—if he pulled out his passport again I was going to strangle him—then finally zipped it up and carefully positioned it under the chair. He straightened up and looked expectantly at me.

I glared at the computer screen while I dialed the interpreter service.

"What is on your mind today," I asked, with about as much warmth and enthusiasm as the overnight techs in radiology usually displayed.

"I was told to come today," he replied.

There wasn't any reason he should have had a follow-up appointment any sooner than one year, but I must have felt guilty about how things had ended the last time so I'd probably overbooked him for an extra appointment just to make him feel better, or maybe to make me feel better. I was disgusted with myself.

In any case, there wasn't anything medical of importance to talk about. His hepatitis wasn't active; his renal cyst was benign. There were no screening tests to discuss. When I told him that I'd canceled his PSA, cholesterol, and colonoscopy tests from the last visit because he'd had them so recently, he simply nodded, taking it in stride without any sort of protest, question, or apology. It was a useless visit. I chided myself for adding to my workload for no good reason.

Then I noticed that the blood pressure written down by the medical assistant was 170/90. I didn't recall him having hypertension, and when I scrolled back to previous visits, I didn't see any abnormal values other than one or two borderline readings of 140/85. I pulled over my sphygmomanometer, conscious of my guilt that I'd forgotten to do a physical exam last time. I took his blood pressure with more care than usual. It was 174/92, high enough to warrant immediate treatment.

I used the interpreter phone to ask if he'd ever had hypertension before. Mr. Ptchetpchdad said no. I asked if any doctor had ever mentioned high blood pressure in the past. He said no.

What an odd thing—a disease just appearing like that, during a medical visit he didn't need. Well, at least it was fortuitous that Mr. Ptchetpchdad was here in the clinic when his blood pressure decided to make its ascent. I started to jot a list of things to do—obtain an immediate EKG, check his electrolytes, evaluate for rare causes of secondary hypertension such as an adrenal tumor, renovascular disease, or a pheochromocytoma.

While I was entering this list into the computer, Mr. Ptchetpchdad said, "My blood pressure only goes up when I think about my daughter who was assassinated."

My mind was still on the hypertension train of thought and several beats went by before I figured out what he'd just said.

"She was seventeen," he said. "They raped her and then they assassinated her."

Slowly, my brain recalibrated from the mundane to the horrifying, as an anvil of silence crushed us. The air grew chilled in the windowless white cube that passes for an office as tears began to seep out of the eyes of the gentleman from Cameroon.

My gaze staggered downward and landed on my desk, where the note from our previous visit was sitting before me. I could see the information under Social History that I'd dutifully typed: *Born in Cameroon, came to US in 2000, married, 5 kids, works in security, no tobacco/ETOH/drugs.*

He hadn't told me anything else at that visit, but then again, why should he have? He was meeting a new doctor. I must have seemed brusque, annoyed, rushed—not exactly a welcoming atmosphere conducive to such revelations.

Mr. Ptchetpchdad pawed at his eyes with thick, rutted fingers to clear the wetness, and I fumbled awkwardly on my desk for tissues. Unable to locate any, I tore open a sterile gauze pad and offered it to him. He took it and hesitantly patted his eyes as though he were unsure whether he wanted the tears to stay or go.

"When?" I finally whispered. "When did this happen?"

"Speak up, Doctor," came a pragmatic voice in the earpiece. "I need to be able to hear you."

I'd completely forgotten about the interpreter.

"When did this happen?" I asked again, embarrassed at having to raise my voice.

"Four months ago."

My fingers stayed numb as I helped Mr. Ptchetpchdad onto the exam table, rechecking his blood pressure for a third time, listening to his heart, running an EKG, and then writing out a prescription for an antihypertensive medication. As I moved mechanically through these actions, my mind went back over our first visit, six weeks ago. All during that visit, while I'd been so irritated at Mr. Ptchetpchdad for not understanding his medical history, for not remembering that he'd had a colonoscopy and a PSA and a cholesterol check and hepatitis C, for making me do unnecessary work, for making me late for my children—all that time there was a fresh memory of his young daughter's assault and murder. His daughter whom he'd had to leave behind in Cameroon when she was nine. His daughter whom he'd been unable to protect.

I wanted to kick myself for being more concerned about efficiency than seeing what was really going on. Of course I couldn't have known of the trauma that he'd experienced, but my response to the confusion about his medical history could have been a discreet probe into other issues rather than annoyance at his usurpation of my time. I had failed my patient.

—❦—

The next morning was a typical one at home—the maelstrom of processing three young children through the necessary morning rituals of washing, dressing, feeding, and preparing for school and day care. I poured all the bowls of cereal, attempting to glance at the newspaper while I slurped down my own breakfast.

Naava wanted the cereal poured first, then the milk. Noah needed the milk poured first, followed by the cereal in carefully calibrated aliquots—something I had to admit was my own quirk as well. Ariel was engaged in expansive postmodern artistic interpretations of her breakfast.

Noah began to wail because he'd gotten a small spoon instead of a big spoon. A fight broke out over who got the orange cup.

"Ariel always gets the orange cup because she's the littlest," Noah said. "I always get stuck with the blue one. It's not fair."

"There's a raisin in my cereal," Naava shrieked. "I hate raisins! You know that."

I did not know that. Last year she loved raisins. The dried-fruit aversion was a recent development.

"I'll take your raisins," Noah said, plunging his fist into Naava's bowl.

"Get your annoying fingers out of my bowl," Naava snapped, whisking her bowl out of his reach, causing a modest tidal wave of cereal over the edge. Juliet sidled up to the table. Her tongue flicked over the edge and scarfed a handful of the overboard flakes.

In the old days, before kids, I used to read the *New York Times* cover to cover each morning, following all the important news items in depth. I didn't leave for work until I was fully abreast of all the major national and international news as well as what was happening in the New York cultural scene and which new books had been favorably reviewed. Now if I was able to extract five minutes each morning to scan the headlines and perhaps read one article or editorial, I felt victoriously connected to the world.

"You poured the *cereal* in my bowl first." Noah moaned, his face welling with tragedy worthy of *La Traviata*. "I wanted the *milk* first. You *never* listen to me."

"Ariel is feeding cereal to Juliet," Naava reported.

"Tattletale," Noah said. Ariel cackled ecstatically as she succeeded in getting Juliet to beg obediently in front of her chair.

I shooed Juliet from the table, retrieved the unwanted raisins, and reversed Noah's milk-cereal order while running my eyes down the front page of the paper. This morning—as it had been for the past few weeks—the news was dominated by the election-related violence in Zimbabwe. Robert Mugabe's ruling party, though obviously the loser in the election, was not prepared to cede its three-decade rule of the country. The spasm of violence against members of the opposition and anyone remotely connected to the voting process was systematically unraveling the country. Today's article was about the murders of family members of opposition politicians and of ordinary people who had voted for the opposition candidate—the wife of a mayor beaten so badly that she could be identified only by the style of braiding in her hair; a suspected opposition supporter killed by dripping bubbles of burning plastic on his naked body; another man whose genitals were strangulated with an elastic band before he was bludgeoned to death. The last one mentioned was a thirty-year-old political organizer who was dragged from bed and garroted in front of his wife and children as they were eating their breakfast porridge.

I eased my spoon back into my bowl, unable to swallow the bite of cereal. I bowed my head over my elbows for a moment as my three children lustily ate their breakfasts in the unfair calm of a Manhattan morning.

"How come Noah gets more napkins?" Naava said. "I want more napkins too."

Ariel submerged her napkin in her bowl and then cleaned the table with it.

"More napkins! More napkins!" Noah cried, imitating Ariel and then flipping his wet napkins into the air. Juliet's tongue made another appearance over the edge of the table, this time snagging the milk-sodden napkins.

I had no idea what sort of turmoil was happening in Cameroon; clearly it didn't rise high enough above the background level of worldwide violence to warrant mention in the *New York Times*.

Nonetheless, they'd raped and murdered a seventeen-year-old. I didn't know who the "they" were in Cameroon, but it didn't really matter. There always seemed to be a "they"—a "they" who could unhinge the social order of a country, a "they" who could plunder and extort, a "they" who could beat Mohammed Ali Amal to a pulp, a "they" who could back a car over Arzouma Érassa's legs, a "they" who could rape Azad Aptekin, a "they" who could pour sulfuric acid down the throat of Samuel Nwanko.

The headline of the article I'd been reading was ONGOING MURDERS IN ZIMBABWE, and the photo showed several bodies lined up on the ground. Now that Naava could read, and Noah was an avid observer, I was much more sensitive about the daily newspaper on our breakfast table. I'd never have envisioned myself as someone who censored what her children read or saw, but now I carefully tucked the front page inside the sports section. There were some things—no matter how truthful—that four- and six-year-olds didn't need to see just yet.

I herded everyone off to brush their teeth. The threat of cavity monsters was the biggest fear in their lives. Right now I was prepared to leave it that way.

As I washed the breakfast dishes, I thought about Thierry Ptchetpchdad and the ultimate impossibility of being able to protect one's children. There'd been many articles recently about the genocide in Darfur, almost mind-numbing in the relentless cruelty they reported, but there was one particular story that I could not shake. A mother and her five children were escaping their hut, which had been torched. The littlest one fell behind, and a Janjaweed soldier casually tossed him into the flames. The mother turned back to pull him out and the soldier told her that if she stepped any closer he'd throw the rest of her children in the fire. It was that moment that refused to release its grip on me—the crystalline horror of it. The mother had no choice but to run off with her four older children as her toddler shrieked her name into the smoke-filled air.

I strapped on everyone's backpack, making sure that Naava had her violin for after-school music lessons, and that Noah had his egg timer for show-and-tell, and that Ariel had her yellow shirt for yellow-shirt day. We spilled noisily out the door, into the elevator, and then out onto the sidewalk. I squeezed their hands tightly as we approached the street, conscious of my urge to hold on to them.

As I dropped them off at day care and school, I was suddenly seized with the fear that I might never see them again. What if today was the day of the deranged gunman? the dirty bomb? the earthquake? the blitzkrieg of Manhattan? What if this last glance of them charging into their classrooms was my last ever?

I elbowed these thoughts out of my head, forcing them to disperse. I would have to live in denial of these horrific possibilities. Although I could not rid myself of the haunting thoughts of the mother in Darfur, of Mr. Ptchetpchdad and his daughter, I would simply have to pretend that this wasn't ever going to happen here in New York. There was no other way to survive.

As I stood there on First Avenue, unsettled by the rapidity with which my children had evaporated from my view, it dawned on me what a luxury denial was. A luxury that allowed us to cope in an irrational world. A luxury that permitted us to impose an order—even an imaginary one—on an unpredictable life. A luxury that Mr. Ptchetpchdad could never again enjoy.

I turned and joined the horde of commuters striding up the avenue. There was a comforting anonymity in the momentum of the crowd. If they had managed to sublimate their existential fears, if they had risked bringing forth their children into the world, if they were moving forward, then I supposed I could too. My first patients would be arriving in five minutes, and I needed to hurry to get to clinic on time. Perhaps my presence in their lives was part of their own effort to sublimate fears—our effort to control their illness an attempt to impose order on their world. Perhaps I was an instrument of their own luxury of denial. There weren't too many luxuries in the world that could be offered, so I'd better not be late.

✐ Chapter Twenty-two ✐

It was Monday after the Thanksgiving weekend. I arrived at clinic a half an hour early to catch up on the backlog of work. My voice mail was flashing with at least ten messages. My mailbox was stuffed with forms for home care, visiting-nurse services, prior authorization for nonformulary medications. I had just gotten through the first two voice messages when there was a knock on the door. It was Samuel Nwanko.

Today he was wearing only sunglasses—no hat, no high collar. His hair was in neat dreadlocks that reached past his ears. He seemed more comfortable than I'd seen him before.

"I was just passing by," he said, "on the way to the SOT office and thought I'd say hello." He still hadn't found a job and still hadn't worked out college enrollment, but he felt that opportunities were available.

"I'm so glad you stopped by, Samuel," I said. "There's actually something I've been meaning to ask you." I paused for a moment to gather my thoughts. Up until now, I'd written about patients only many years after our encounters, sometimes only after a patient's death, or long after I'd ceased to be their physician. My first books had involved reaching far back into the past of memories and recollections. But now, as writing took up a larger role in my life, I decided that if I wanted to write about patients I'd have to approach them in real time. I'd have to get their permission, perhaps even interview them—outside of our regular contact. I'd never done this before, and I had mixed emotions about the propriety. But I'd decided that I would be straightforward.

"Samuel," I said, "in addition to being a doctor, I also do some writing. I usually write about patients who've had a powerful impact on me, and whose stories might help future doctors." I stopped again to organize my thoughts. Something about the public acknowledgment of this made me feel awkward, even a little ashamed. "I was wondering if I could write about your story. Please don't feel obliged—"

He put up a hand to cut me off before I could even finish. "I think I would like to tell my story," he said. "I have actually been trying to write it myself, but I am not getting very far." He reached up to push a dreadlock past his shoulder. I could see the pink scars on his wrists. "Ask me any questions you want. But then I will think about it, before you publish it."

I nodded in agreement, thankful that I had a half hour before the first patient was scheduled. Samuel began to tell me about his childhood in Imo State, and what it was like growing up as a pastor's son. When we got to the part about starting college, I asked him what year he had matriculated.

"You know," he said, embarrassed at his forgetfulness, "I can't even remember. That shows you how much my brain has been through." He reached into his back pocket and pulled out his wallet. From the wallet he extracted his student ID card and bent his head toward the fine print. "It was 2003," he said. "September 2003."

From where I was sitting, I could not see the details of the card. But I could see that there was a photo. A "before" photo. I had no idea what he'd looked like before the attack, and it had never occurred to me to ask. But now this card was in the air between us. I was pained by an uncomfortable feeling that maybe I was pressing too much, that I was digging deeper than was appropriate. Was this the doctor in me or the writer in me that wanted to see the photo? Perhaps I needed to stop here.

Then Samuel placed the card on the desk and wordlessly slid it over to me. I didn't recognize the face, but I hadn't expected to. What struck me most was the difference in skin color. When I'd first met Samuel Nwanko, I assumed that the dark black color of his skin was his natural color; the pink and white were the scars from the acid. But I was wrong. The black too had been scar. The young man in this photo had light brown skin. His eyes were almond shaped, nose narrow; his lips were straight and smooth, seeming on the verge of smiling. A soft corona of dark hair surrounded the handsome face. I closed my eyes briefly, and the haunting melody of the Vivaldi cello sonata edged into my head. I thanked him and slid the card back.

By the time Samuel left, my morning patients were already registered and waiting. It wasn't until after lunch that I was able to finish
sorting through my voice mail. There were three more prescription requests from pharmacies, another home-care agency needing
medical authorization. And then a weak, raspy, but familiar voice
came through on the machine: "It's your patient Juan Moreno. I've
been in the hospital for over a week and nobody has come to see
me."

I'd known that Mr. Moreno was due for an elective overnight
admission for his AICD, but I hadn't known the exact date of the
procedure. I'd assumed I would be informed somehow. I'd be called
to provide preoperative clearance or I'd need to order labs for him
or fill out forms or something.

Evidently not.

Then it hit me what he'd said: "in the hospital for over a week."
AICDs normally take one day. Something bad must have happened.

I dashed up to the seventeenth floor and collared the intern taking care of him. The holiday weekend had been at the end of the
month-long rotation, and the previous team had probably figured
that the new team would call me, and the new team probably figured that the old team had called me.

It was partially my fault: I could have been more assiduous in
calling to find out when his AICD was scheduled, but the accepted
etiquette was that the inpatient doctors had the responsibility of
informing the outpatient doctors, who might not have any other
way to know what was happening.

The intern reported to me that the AICD had been successfully
placed in Mr. Moreno's chest last week and it had been expected
that he'd return home the next day. The AICD was primed to sit
quietly in his chest doing nothing unless Mr. Moreno suffered a
life-threatening arrhythmia, such as ventricular tachycardia or ventricular fibrillation. Then and only then would it deliver a shock.
But for some reason, the AICD had begun to fire here and there
during Mr. Moreno's normal atrial-fibrillation rhythm. Each time
it fired, it was like a surprise karate chop to the chest.

At every shock, Mr. Moreno was thrown into a panic, convinced he was about to die. He grew terrified of the prospect of an unexpected shock. He began to limit his activity, avoiding anything he thought might precipitate a shock. Now he was a hospital agoraphobe, scared even to move from his bed.

His atrial fibrillation had begun beating at a higher rate than it ever had. The cardiologists were loading on one medication after another but none seemed to control the rapid rate. Each medication had side effects—constipation, nausea, edema, drowsiness, headache—and Mr. Moreno managed to get them all.

When I entered Juan Moreno's room, I was shocked by how looked. His eyes were sunken into puffy lids, his face blanched of color. This 280-pound bear of a man had been rendered slack, forlorn. I realized that in our fifteen years together, Mr. Moreno had never once been hospitalized, despite his formidable list of medical conditions. I'd never actually seen him in the humbling hospital gown, with the ill-fitting slippers, forcibly supine in a hospital bed, raked by the limp fluorescent light. The desperate look of illness on his face was more than I could bear.

But when I walked into the room, Mr. Moreno struggled to pull himself up and then announced proudly to his three other roommates, "*This* is my doctor." Then he paused and corrected himself. "No, she is no my doctor; she is my *sister*. She is like family to me."

His praise made me feel awkward, and not just because I was embarrassed that for a whole week I hadn't known he was in the hospital. What made me feel most awful was that Mr. Moreno was sitting here in this hospital bed suffering all these adverse outcomes because I had convinced him to get the AICD.

But now everything was a mess. Nobody could explain why the AICD was firing so wantonly. When tested with an external monitor, the device appeared to be working fine. AICD shocks could be so painful that many patients were sure they were dying; many even experienced a form of posttraumatic stress disorder from the fright. Mr. Moreno was so scared of the shocks that he was willing to put up with the humiliation of a bedside commode rather than risk the ten steps to the bathroom. For most of his waking hours, he simply cowered under his sheets.

"Before this, I feel fine. I do all things I want to do," he said, barely able to muster up enough voice for outrage. "But now I too scared to take any steps because that thing will fire at me. And now I have twice as many pills as when I started!"

He felt duped by the cardiologists. The cardiologists from the clinic who had so strongly urged the AICD didn't ever come see him in the hospital. The ones in the hospital kept piling on new medications and proposing new settings for the AICD, but Mr. Moreno became frustrated with the entire process. He wasn't necessarily angry that the AICD didn't work as we'd hoped—he had a broad enough vision to accept the imperfections of life—he was mainly angry about how his body had been battered by the process. He had lost complete faith in the cardiologists' care. After eleven days in the hospital—angry, bitter, and weakened—Mr. Moreno insisted that they turn off the AICD and send him home.

To me, it was the worst imaginable outcome: Here was a man who had been doing well enough in his life, despite his many medical conditions—able to do everything he needed to do. Then we doctors convinced him to get a prophylactic treatment for an arrhythmia that he'd never yet had. He came out of the procedure feeling sicker and weaker than when he'd started. And now, with the AICD turned off, he couldn't even obtain the benefit of the device should a grave arrhythmia occur.

There is no free lunch, I always told my students, even for the simplest medical intervention like an aspirin or a blood draw or an X-ray. Everything had a cost, a risk, a side effect, a harm. And now one of my dearest patients, the one who'd been with me the longest in my medical career and who trusted me unreservedly, was on the receiving end of the costliest, sourest lunch.

When Mr. Moreno showed up in my clinic, one week after his discharge, he looked as though he'd aged a decade. He stared at the floor with hooded eyes, and his words came in weary, sibilant fragments. "Before this, I am fine. Now, I am sick man." His cane was now a necessity, no longer just for show. "I can't take two steps out of my house."

He was depressed and embittered; not one positive thing had come from the ordeal. With his ever gracious and generous attitude, however, Mr. Moreno was fastidious about not blaming me. I knew that I wasn't responsible for the cardiologists' behavior, and of course the malfunctioning device was not anyone's fault, but I shared some of the responsibility for this mess. Even though it was Mr. Moreno who'd signed the consent form, I was the one, in the end, who had made the decision to do the procedure.

"This summer we planned to go to Puerto Rico," he mumbled into his lap. "How can I go now? I am old, sick man." He seemed so depressed that I considered prescribing antidepressant medications.

I apologized profusely for what had happened. I told him that I could understand if he no longer trusted his care here. At that he looked up, indignant. "Bellevue saved my life, way back in the beginning, and you my best doctor, so I never leave Bellevue."

I was impressed at his continued dedication to Bellevue. I was grateful for this but despondent at what the situation had wrought. Mr. Moreno was a changed man, and I worried that we might have permanently damaged him.

❧ Chapter Twenty-three ❧

Two weeks later, as I walked from the elevator to the clinic for my morning patient session, I saw Jade Collier in the waiting room. She was talking to a fellow in a wheelchair, the armrests of their chairs nearly overlapping. "Take another patient before me," she said, waving me cheerily away. "Eduardo and I have some things to work on."

I hadn't even booted up the computer in my office when the clerk called from the front desk. "There's a patient here, someone from the SOT program. He doesn't have an appointment but needs to talk to you. He says that it's very important. Can I send him over to you?"

A minute later, Arzouma Érassa, the gentleman from Togo, opened my door and poked his head in. "Forgive me for interrupting," he said, stumbling over his words, "but it is so very, very important."

I beckoned him in and he perched himself on the edge of the seat, his arms and legs seeming to quiver with electricity. He shifted three times in the seat, and then finally crossed his arms and legs to rein in the motion.

"It is my wife," Mr. Érassa said, not waiting for me to dial the interpreter.

There was only a fraction of a second of pause after he spoke, but in that fraction of a second my mind raced through the likely possibilities—she was being held hostage in the jungles of Togo; she'd been raped by rebels; she'd been arrested by the authorities; she'd been caught in crossfire; her house had been burned; she'd been tortured because of her husband's activities.

"My wife," he said again. "She is to arrive next month. We finally have visa." And then a capacious smile bloomed across his face. His elation settled over us like the sun-drenched scent from a freshly laundered sheet lofted in the air. One of the rare moments of joy in the SOT program.

Mr. Érassa still had nightmares about burned bodies and spilling intestines, but they had lessened a bit. He was eager to find an apartment—he'd been sharing a room up until now—but wasn't sure if the salary from his security job would permit this.

"But most important," he said, his limbs slipping out from where he'd corralled them, "is appointment for gynecologist." His arms and legs began to bob like they were independently wired. "We will try for baby again and she must see doctor soon."

Although his wife wasn't with him at our visit, or even yet in the country, I provided a referral for her to the gynecology clinic accompanied by a letter explaining the special circumstances. It seemed like there was no time to waste.

I finished with my next patient, then called in Jade Collier. I thought about her history as I waited for her to wheel herself from the far end of the waiting room. It had been nearly forty years since that dive in Brookfield River, eighteen years since she'd moved to the United States. Jade was the only patient I knew who'd immigrated with a significant preexisting disability, who'd navigated the vast bureaucracy without the ability to be invisible or to blend into the crowd. I wondered how much of an impediment the wheelchair had been in this process.

I asked Jade about the wheelchair when she got to my office.

"Actually," she said, shaking out her wrists, "the wheelchair brings out the nicer side of people. People on the street—New Yorkers, mind you!—make eye contact, smile, say hello. And people are always trying to help. This is great when I'm stuck at a curb without a ramp. Sometimes I don't actually need the help, but I let them help me anyway because I think it might hurt their feelings if I said no."

"What's the worst thing?" I asked.

"It's about sex," she said, chuckling. "That's all everybody wants to know—can I feel it? Even total strangers will ask. When I was younger I used to try to avoid the question." She leaned over the edge of the chair and scrunched her face. "Now I say, 'None of your effin' business!'"

We rolled up her pants and checked her legs for swelling. Edema could be hard to control if the muscles of the legs weren't helping to pump the blood back up to the heart. Jade's edema wasn't too bad today. "I keep the legs elevated whenever possible," she said, "but sometimes that's just plain awkward."

"Do you ever think of returning to New Zealand?" I asked as we finished the physical exam.

"Waiting on the green card," she said, pulling out her leather biking gloves from her bag. "Can't leave the country till it's re- solved, but it's taking years and years." She slipped one glove on. "I'm in a slight bit of limbo because I originally came on a church worker's visa. Then after a few years, the church went and moved its office to the second floor. There was no elevator, so my job sput- tered out." She gave a shrug and then pulled on the other glove.

As I entered the details of Jade's visit into the computer, I thought about the popular image of illegal immigrants and how it rested heavily on the perceived ability of immigrants to secrete themselves in society's shadows. This, in turn, relied on good health. To sneak across a desert—like Julia Barquero did—walking for weeks on end during the night, outrunning border police, is something that only the young and the able-bodied can do. Had it not been for the bad cardiac luck conferred by her genetics, Julia could easily have spent her life doing the labor that nobody else wanted to do or see or even acknowledge—scrubbing bathrooms and offices at night. She could have lived her life quietly in the dark shadows of America.

But it wasn't as easy to be invisible in a wheelchair. One couldn't outrun a border guard or take a less expensive apartment in a fifth- floor walk-up. Most jobs available to those without papers involved physical labor and were unlikely to be wheelchair accessible.

Ordinary day-to-day travel involved a great deal of visibility. There was the option of the public bus, in which all the passengers had to wait—sometimes impatiently—as the stairs were converted to an elevator-type platform, the seats pushed up to make room for the wheelchair, the wheelchair secured in place. Or there was the option of Access-A-Ride service, which involved applications, interviews, and recertification every five years.

But this visibility seemed to suit Jade Collier. Neither disability nor immigration status were things that needed to be hidden. In fact, she'd become a Big Apple Greeter—a volunteer who stepped out into the bright light to welcome visitors to New York City. She could show them the sights of New York as only a local could, with an insider's knowledge of which subway stops were wheelchair-accessible, which restaurants had wide bathrooms, and where to charge up an electric chair when you were out and about for the day.

When we'd finished our visit, Jade leaned over and whispered to me about the young man I'd seen her with in the waiting room. "Eduardo couldn't get his socks on. Sometimes the littlest things are the most important."

Indeed.

—◦◦◦◦—

Dr. Chan was in for a blood-pressure check. He had been doing well over the past two years—his pressure and diabetes were staying controlled. His wife's Alzheimer's disease had progressed but only incrementally. Mrs. Geng was home today with her attendant.

"Everybody in waiting room... speak Spanish," he said while I pumped up the blood-pressure cuff. "I must learn... Cervantes, no?"

I smiled as the manometer clicked downward, recording 142/70. "If I could ever get to the level of reading Cervantes," I said, "my job would be a lot easier."

"But more Chinese than Spanish people," he replied. "You need learn Mandarin now."

As I wrote out his antihypertensive prescriptions, Dr. Chan and I continued our discussion about the many different immigrants at Bellevue Hospital. I mentioned to him that I was interested in the stories of immigrants and that I was interviewing some to learn about their experiences in the American health-care system. Dr. Chan immediately proposed that we meet to talk and that we do it the very next day.

The next day at the appointed time I walked across the street from my apartment building to his. Dr. Chan was waiting for me in the community room armed with a red plastic bag that contained a thermos of tea, two glass cups, napkins, and a package of Chinese cookies. He carefully arranged the provisions on the Formica table.

His arthritic hands struggled with the packaging—the cookies were individually wrapped—but he graciously acceded when I offered to help.

Dr. Chan told me that he had been born in a small city in the southeastern Fujian Province. Both his father and grandfather had graduated from college and worked as teachers. His father married three times. Dr. Chan's first mother—his biological mother—died of tuberculosis. His second mother died of cholecystitis shortly after her marriage. His third mother was not formally educated but had taught herself, reading voraciously any books that crossed the threshold of the Chan home.

Of the four children in the family, one became an engineer, another became a chemist, and two became physicians. Dr. Chan trained as a cardiologist, eventually becoming the vice president of the main public hospital, though he also remained an active clinician, spending long hours treating patients. He'd published books and articles about the pulmonary effects of cardiac disease. "I was...very famous doctor...in China," he said mildly. He told me that whenever he got on the bus, scores of patients would recognize and greet him.

His own children succeeded just as well as his siblings—two engineers, one businessman, one physician, all still living in China. Dr. Chan told me that the Cultural Revolution hadn't affected him much because he'd worked in a public hospital treating peasants and politicians alike.

He conceded that life was good in New York—political stability, more freedoms, reliable supplies of food and goods—even though financially he and Mrs. Geng were just barely scraping by. He was extremely proud that he and his wife had finally achieved American citizenship, a process that had been arduous and protracted. But Dr. Chan said that his life had also been good in China—he had his children, his relatives, and a healthy dose of community respect. In New York he was just another elderly Chinese immigrant. Still, he added, "New York is...our home. This is where...we stay."

Dr. Chan thanked me profusely for this house call. "I must now...prepare lunch," he said, rising slowly with the aid of his cane. "My wife...always hungry in...midmorning." He gathered up the thermos of tea and offered me the rest of the cookies to take home for my children.

I watched him shuffle toward the elevator, the red plastic shopping bag dangling from his wrist. In some ways, Dr. Chan represented the immigrant success story. Despite physical, financial, and language challenges, he'd managed to create a decent life for himself and his wife. He'd successfully navigated the byzantine immigration system, obtaining green cards and then citizenship for both of them. He'd managed to find them adequate housing and obtain Medicaid coverage—he and his wife would not suffer the risks of being homeless or uninsured. He'd been able to arrange for a home attendant to assist them—he and his wife would not suffer the debility of sickness in isolation. All this from a man who was ninety years old, who weighed about ninety pounds, whose voice was barely louder than a dragonfly's. Julia Barquero and Amadou Sow—though both younger by half a century—hadn't been able to match Dr. Chan's achievement of green card and citizenship, and now they were paying for it with their health.

I crossed the street back to my building, contemplating the prodigious effort required for all the things Dr. Chan achieved. How did he fill out forms with his limited English from a Shakespeare class? How did he wait on long lines with his rickety wooden cane? How did he battle voice-mail systems? Deal with impatient clerical staff? Jump through endless bureaucratic hoops? I envisioned myself trying to negotiate housing, health insurance, home care in a foreign country, in a foreign language, in a frail state. It would never happen; I'd be found dead in my hovel within weeks.

Quiet, unassuming Dr. Chan—red-blooded American hero. The kind of guy who should be on a postage stamp, I thought. This was the type of person I'd tell my children to emulate. The type of man—like those in my grandparents' generation—who was brave enough to emigrate into the unknown with few resources and succeed in creating a new life. I thought about my generation— wusses all! We couldn't hold a candle to Dr. Chan or our own grandparents.

I dodged a taxi to make it to the other side of the street, then climbed the steps to my building. I'd do some Googling when I got home: I was going to figure out how to nominate someone for a stamp. All I needed was Dr. Chan's portrait. Perhaps the postal service would make an exception and would photograph Dr. Chan and Mrs. Geng together. That would be fitting: the model Americans.

Chapter Twenty-four

Nazma Uddin was on the schedule for an appointment, but Azina—now a freshman at a community college in Queens—showed up instead. Mrs. Uddin wasn't feeling well and had sent her daughter to pick up her prescriptions. The elevators were packed, so Azina had sprinted up the three flights of stairs in order to be on time. She was breathless when she arrived—skin flushed, cheeks puffing from exertion, upper lip peaked with moisture. Her hair was coming undone from its ponytail. It was only when she used the back of her hand to wipe off the sweat that it occurred to me what was different: there was no veil and no head scarf. Her round cherubic face was completely exposed. The thick strands of her dark hair were glistening even under the harsh fluorescent lights. She wore jeans and a sweater; no gown covered her clothes.

"I'm sorry my mom couldn't make it," she said, taking quick breaths between words. "She promises not to miss the next appointment." She pulled a clutch of refill slips out of her bag. "These are the prescriptions that she needs."

"Azina," I said, my mouth hanging open, "what happened to…" Then I stopped, unsure if I was treading on territory that might be too personal. Had Azina embarked on a college rebellion? Was there a falling-out with her family? Did she find a boyfriend who was less religious? Was she making a statement about assimilation?

But then I recalled how forthrightly and warmly Azina had spoken about her veil the other time, and so I decided to ask. "Azina, what happened to your veil?"

Azina laid the papers on my desk and smoothed them carefully. Her breathlessness was receding and she spoke more slowly now. "I, uh, I had an incident three days ago."

"An incident?" I said. "What do you mean?"

"I was waiting for the bus, on my way to school, and there was this guy at the bus stop." Azina looked past me as she spoke, directing her words toward the wall. "He was looking at me funny, then he started to talk to me. 'The attack on 9/11 was your fault,' he said. 'You killed three thousand Americans.' So I said to him, 'I'm Bangladeshi. Bangladesh had nothing to do with 9/11.'

"Then he started to walk toward me in this threatening way, saying over and over, 'It was your fault—9/11 was your fault.' I backed up against the wall of the bus shelter and then he pulled out a knife and waved it in my face. 'You people ruined our country,' he yelled. I couldn't move. He had me pinned against the wall. Then he reached over with the knife and tore off my veil and head scarf with it. I was so scared he was going to stab me. The only thing I remember was that the pins that held it in the back scratched my neck as the veil came off. I must have screamed—I don't even remember—and some teenagers passing by jumped on him and pulled him off me."

Azina's voice sounded wooden as she spoke, but to me it was a sledgehammer in the chest. "Someone called the cops," she continued, "and they came pretty quickly. But I felt so naked, so exposed, in front of all these strangers, so embarrassed that I was the cause of all this. The police brought me home. They tried to make me feel safe. A detective came over the next day to get all the details, but I wouldn't leave the house for two whole days. Today—today's the first day I've gone out. My father told me to stop wearing the veil, that it was too dangerous."

I looked up at Azina, her somber demeanor a punishing contrast to the voluble, engaging teenager who'd spoken to me last time. I reached over and touched her sleeve. "Azina, I'm so sorry this happened. This shouldn't—"

Azina cut me off. "It's okay," she said. "It's not anyone's fault. There are stupid people everywhere and he was just a stupid person."

"But still," I said, "this is a horrible..."

"I'm getting over it," she said, the color returning to her voice. "I've decided that I will probably wear my head scarf, but maybe not the veil. My father is against it, but this is America and I can do what I want. Besides, I can't sit around feeling sorry for myself. I need my energy to finish pharmacy school and to take care of my mother." She rolled her eyes dramatically. "And you know how much TLC my mother needs!"

A week later, I had a new patient—Qayyid Bassam. After introducing myself, I asked him where he was from. "Yemen," he told me. I was suddenly overcome with a feeling that was hard to describe. Despite my many years at Bellevue, I'd never had a patient from Yemen, and now a powerful sense of connection arose. Somebody from my grandparents' country!

We addressed all of Mr. Bassam's medical issues—mild psoriasis, an inguinal hernia—but then we had a long discussion about Yemen. He told me that he was from Ta'izz, but also had family in Sana'a. He'd come to America about the same year I'd started medical school, had married a Yemenite woman and had four children here.

I told him that my paternal grandfather came from the city of Afar; Afari, or Ofri, identifies the residents of Afar. He and his sister—young children at the time—had ridden in the saddlebags of a camel as the entire community made the pilgrimage on foot through Saudi Arabia to Palestine.

Mr. Bassam peppered me with questions and I told him the stories that my father had shared with me. The Jews of Yemen apparently began returning to Israel in 1881 because of a famous verse in the book of Solomon—*Amarti e'eleh b'tamar*. It translated to "I said I will climb up into the date-palm tree" but was taken to mean "going up" to the land of Israel. The numerical value of the Hebrew letters of this phrase added up to 642, so in the Jewish year 5642 (1881), the Yemenite Jews began their migration home.

My *saba* arrived in Palestine during the waning years of the Ottoman Empire. He grew up to become a floor-layer and eventually built a house for his wife and five children in the Kerem HaTemanim, the ramshackle Yemenite neighborhood in Tel Aviv. This was the house where we stayed—decades later—when my father brought our family on summer visits; I always slept on the closet-size back terrace. I still had crisp recollections of hanging laundry on the roof with my *safta*, peering out at the raucous open-air *shuk* on the next block and the corner food stands where old Yemenite men gathered to eat steaming bowls of *fuul*. Over the

years, this slum transmogrified into a gentrified Tel Aviv neighborhood, but it still maintained a solid core of old-time Yemenites, the
ones who claimed to speak the purest Hebrew because their tribe
had left Israel during the time of the Second Temple and had kept
the language free from outside influence during the intervening centuries. To this day, Yemenite Jews consider themselves distinct from
Sephardic and Ashkenazi Jews.

Mr. Bassam spread his hands expansively. "In two years I will
bring my children to Yemen for a visit, and I invite you and your
family to join us. You will be a guest in our home." He went on
to tell me how Jews had always lived safely in Yemen and were
always welcomed. I knew that the historical record reflected a de-
cidedly more mixed picture, but it was indeed true that there were
long periods in which Jews lived comfortably in Arab countries,
many generations in which the similarities of these Middle Eastern
cultures rather than the differences ruled the day. I was genuinely
moved by his gesture.

Mr. Bassam touched my shoulder and then brought his hand
to his chest. "You and I, we are cousins." I was reminded of
Mohammed Khalil and how his warm embrace of our religions
had put my hesitations to shame. "We are from the same family,"
Mr. Bassam continued. "My children will host your children and
we will travel home together to our country."

Our country. Even though I had enough maternal mix of Eastern
European background in me to make me a mongrel, there was
something undeniably uplifting about being included in this sweeping Semitic concept. I was, after all, walking around with a Yemeni-
derived name and a full paternal set of Yemeni-derived genes. I'd
never referred to Yemen as "my country," but Mr. Bassam made me
feel like a legitimate member.

At the end of my visit with Mr. Bassam, I handed him his prescriptions and appointments. He scribbled his cell phone number
on a piece of paper and pressed it toward me. "When you need
jachnun, zhug, olives, dates, *shakshouka*—you call me. I know
where to get the best and I will bring to you." I remembered my
safta serving me *shakshouka*—eggs with spicy stewed tomatoes—
the year I'd announced I was vegetarian.

"*Salaam aleikum,*" I said as we shook hands, thinking that I'd better start learning more Arabic. I'd have to ask my father for some useful phrases.

"*Aleikum salaam,*" Mr. Bassam replied with a small bow. As he walked out the door, he turned and offered again, "*Hilbah, malawach, fuul*—whatever you need—I bring the best." Then he winked at me. "Only the Yemenites know where to get the best."

～ Chapter Twenty-five ～

Mohammed Ali Amal returned for a second visit. He greeted me politely and somberly, as he had last time. "You cured my restless legs," he said, bowing slightly at the torso, "and I wish to thank you." Apparently the gabapentin had worked. A minor victory, but its joy quickly dissipated.

"America is like a prison," he said when I asked him how he was doing. His head angled downward, chin against his chest. The bridge of his cheeks and his nose seemed to cast a penumbra of sorrow over his face. "I almost wish I'd never started the asylum process." This was a statement I'd never heard before. Most clients of the SOT program were eager to pursue political asylum, despite the frustrations involved. For most, it was their holy grail, and they devoted their full resources to it.

"You don't want political asylum?" I asked, incredulous.

"It's not worth it," he replied, an undercurrent of anger gathering in his voice. "While the papers are in process, I cannot leave this country. At least in Jordan, I had friends, contacts, a community. When I left Jordan to come to America, I lost my legal residency there and so can't go back." He stared down at his polished leather shoes. "America is a prison that I can't escape."

Mr. Amal's only adventure in America—a trip to a computer trade show in Las Vegas—was an unmitigated disaster. A fellow Arab—a man from Syria—approached him at a casino and befriended him. Somehow he convinced Mr. Amal to loan him a few dollars to play the slot machine. Things happened quickly, and the man managed to lose three hundred dollars of Mr. Amal's money. "Wait here," the man had said, "I'll get my money to pay you back." Mr. Amal waited for an hour and the man never showed.

The only moment of levity came when Mr. Amal said, with completely genuine puzzlement, "But how did he know I was an Arab?"

When I said, "Well, you don't look Irish," he smiled for the first time.

On this four-day trip he'd managed to have two car accidents.

The first, he told me, was a true accident: a bird flew into the window and he slammed on the brakes, getting rear-ended by the car behind him. But the second related to Iraq. He'd been pulling out of a parking spot when he saw someone standing to his left. He turned to say "Good afternoon" to the person and was flooded with a recollection of waiting in line at the checkpoint to enter Iraq on that ill-fated visit to his family.

There'd been a long line of cars at that checkpoint, and when he finally arrived at the front he turned to the soldier standing outside his window on the left. "Good afternoon," he'd said. "How does this day find you?" He remembered how the soldier's face transformed from a taut militaristic expression to a hesitant smile. The soldier relaxed his grip on his automatic rifle.

"Thank you, my friend," the soldier had replied, leaning forward toward the open car window, looking like the ordinary family man that he probably was. "Your greeting has warmed my day." It was a throwback to the old Iraq, the Iraq of courtesy and politeness, the Iraq before the war.

There were many other flashbacks from that visit to Iraq; this was the only one that didn't involve blood. Perhaps it was the connection to what Mr. Amal loved about his homeland that made this flashback so potent. Perhaps it was the poignant flicker of civility before the brutality. Whatever it was, it was enough to distract him in Las Vegas, and he sheared the side of his rental car against a concrete wall. The rental agency held him financially responsible for the damages.

While he was visiting the crowded booths in the cavernous exhibition hall, his laptop was stolen. "I put my bag down for a second," he said, "because I needed to get a business card for one of those raffles. It was only a second, but the laptop was gone." By the end of his trip his cell phone had disappeared too. "That one, maybe I lost it," he said, dropping his palms in resignation. "My brain is so scattered."

Mr. Amal had stopped attending the SOT program. "I feel awkward attending a program that's free. It's not right that I don't pay."

This was another statement that I'd never heard before. No one had ever complained about lack of cost as a problem. In the face of all he'd experienced, his sense of rectitude and decency was impressive. I thought about the massive fund-raising efforts the program organizers struggled with. "You could," I said tentatively, "make a donation. You don't have to, but it is a charitable organization that accepts donations."

"I'd like that," he said, the tense muscles of his cheekbones quivering.

On a lark, I asked him if he'd ever been to Kalustyan's, a Middle Eastern/Indian food store three blocks from Bellevue in the section of Murray Hill that had unofficially been named Curry Hill. In a few jam-packed cubic feet, Kalustyan's stocked every possible food—spicy curries from Thailand, frozen appetizers from Egypt, six types of garam masala from India, olives from Israel, red pepper sauce from Algeria, lentils from Pakistan, cultured yogurt drinks from Jordan. The second floor was crammed with cookware—*idli* cookers for making the savory lentil patties, titanium *tadka* pans for heating spice mixtures, wooden *chakla* boards, *ibrik* coffeepots for making Turkish coffee, stainless steel *thali* platters, stone mortars and pestles, aluminum *kadai* woks, Middle Eastern glass tea sets, copper *nargilas*. In the corner was a miniature deli presided over by a tiny white-haired Armenian Jordanian man who pressed spoonfuls of his heavenly vegetable soup on all those who waited on line for his world-famous *mujadarra* sandwiches. Kalustyan's was so popular that the city designated its street frontage as an official taxi stop so that taxi drivers could rest for fifteen minutes and stock up on foods from home. "It's not my area of medical expertise," I said, "but I recommend you wander in there. No one ever leaves Kalustyan's empty-handed."

We stood up at the end of the visit and shook hands. As I opened the door to show him out, he reminded me to give him the donation information for the SOT program. I handed him the papers and watched as he disappeared from sight. The air hardly rippled in his wake.

Twenty-four hours after I watched Mr. Amal slip out the door, I watched my cello teacher slip two photocopied sheets of paper from his bag and smooth them onto my music stand. The moment had finally arrived. After three years of sweating through etudes, scales, and simplified excerpts, it was time to start the Bach suites.

The six unaccompanied cello suites by Bach are iconic in the repertoire. The first suite is the most famous and has been overplayed almost to the point of sentimental kitsch. But like other overplayed works—Vivaldi's *Four Seasons* and Mozart's *Eine kleine Nachtmusik*—the underlying music is still spectacular, no matter how often it's been dredged up for movies, TV commercials, and cell phone ringtones. To listen to it again may feel overly familiar. But to play it—well, that was another matter entirely. It was an opportunity, as a doctor-musician colleague once put it, to "touch the hem of that greatness."

Monday afternoons with SOT patients were daunting. The breadth of brutality of human beings never ceased to astound. The energy, effort, and creativity invested in destroying the human body and spirit seemed limitless. What sort of response could I offer that was meaningful in the face of such overwhelming trauma?

No matter what I said or did with my SOT patients, it always felt useless. It was a different feeling of uselessness than I felt, for example, with a patient dying of cancer. Disease—no matter how painful or humiliating or even self-inflicted—was something that occurred. Disease utilized intransitive verbs.

But torture was transitive—done by somebody to somebody. Having a leg amputated because of complications from diabetes wasn't the same as having it hacked off by a machete. I felt as though I had something in my clinical repertoire to offer the diabetic who faced amputation of a foot. But I was at a complete loss for the Sierra Leonean whose arms had been macheteed off.

It wasn't just because there were medical treatments for the diabetic to prevent the next amputation, but that diabetes was an entity separate from oneself and didn't have a face. Nobody *did* diabetes to anyone—the disease just occurred.

Torture, on the other hand, had a face. Somebody, an actual person, did it. A human being raised the knife, poured the acid, heaved the boot, set the fire, inflicted the rape. And that, I think, was what made these patient encounters so unsettling, above and beyond contemplating the horror that the victim himself had endured. *Somebody* did this, some member of our humanity, and, whether I liked it or not, I was part of that same humanity.

The sheet music of the first Bach suite appeared straightforward—two pages of evenly spaced notes in the key of G. No intricate timing, no double-sharps, no key changes, no clef shifts, no fancy ornamentation. But as anyone who has ever tussled with Bach knows, that simplicity is ruthlessly deceptive. "One measure at a time," my teacher instructed me. "It needs to be completely memorized. Expect to put in at least a year on this." This was said without irony.

Week after week, month after month, I tiptoed gingerly through the music. I found myself focusing ever more narrowly on a single page, a single line, a single measure—even a single note. Temperamentally, this was the exact opposite of the din of meaningless minutiae that clattered the halls of the hospital. All efforts here needed to be focused on struggling to achieve precisely the right note.

But then there was a step even beyond that. The note didn't merely have to be right—it also had to be beautiful. Beauty gets short shrift in medicine. Beauty is inherently unpragmatic—it doesn't enhance efficiency, increase productivity, earn a grant, or cure a patient. But it feels necessary. When I'd survived a measure and could play several notes in sequence, the beauty was astounding—the type of beauty that really did take the breath away.

I sometimes felt as though I had to stack up Vivaldi, Lully, and Bach against Mugabe, Hussein, bin Laden, and all the random dictators who littered the globe. There had to be a counterbalance in this world, a counterbalance that was both metaphorical and actual. To live in this world, to accept that such cruelty was a reality, I had to know that beauty was an equal reality. Even if some humans seemed to exist solely to offer pain and destruction, there were others who existed only to create beauty. The chance to feel the hem of that beauty graze the cheek—even fleetingly—was sometimes the only thing that kept the last straw at bay.

∽ Chapter Twenty-six ∽

Three months after the terrible AICD episode, Juan Moreno was back in my office. The color had largely returned to his face, though maybe it was just redness from the icy winter day. He still used the cane, but he didn't lean on it as heavily. His depression had dissipated somewhat, but there remained a distinct strand of bitterness in his mien.

"Do you know what they want to do now?" he said to me with a pained look of resignation. "They want to go back in. They want to put in a new box and cut some of the connections in my heart. They say it will solve my problems."

Mr. Moreno's residual problems—the atrial fibrillation rate that was difficult to control, and the useless metal box sitting inside of him, doing nothing but taking up space—could possibly be solved by an ablation.

The cardiologists wanted to ablate the electrical pathways running from the atria of his heart to the ventricles. Although the atria would still be in fibrillation, the ventricles—the chambers that did the actual pumping of the blood—would no longer receive these abnormal signals and so would not race.

However, once the atria were cut off from the ventricles, a pacemaker would have to tell the ventricles to pump. This pacemaker could be set at a sedate, even rate. This would relieve Mr. Moreno of the tyranny of a rapid, irregular heart rate, and he could probably stop taking many of the medications we were giving him to control the rate.

The original AICD would be replaced with one that would, presumably, work correctly and also do pacemaker duty. However, the ablation and AICD-pacemaker placement was another invasive procedure.

"I don't want more things in my heart," he said, pressing his hand against his chest. "But if you tell me I need it, I do it."

Once again I tried to solicit Mr. Moreno's opinions on the pros and cons of the procedure, and again he simply replied that he'd do whatever I told him. Only this time, the words came out tinged with resignation, maybe even regret.

I looked over at Mr. Moreno. The soft folds of his neck sat like a cushion between his head and torso. His generously rounded cheeks pushed his eyes up into a friendly squint. Scattered hairs poked up in a faint corona around his scalp. Liver spots dotted the backs of his hands, which lay crossed atop the curve of his cane. I knew just about every detail of his face, and he probably knew all the details of mine. He and I had been gazing at each other across the corner of my desk for about a third of my lifetime and about a quarter of his.

I sat back and contemplated our longevity. Mr. Moreno had known me as an intern, then as a resident. He waited patiently when I took time to travel after residency. He was excited to learn that I was getting married. He put up, good-naturedly, with two maternity leaves and then my sabbatical in Costa Rica. Similarly, I'd followed the trajectory of Mr. Moreno's second parenthood with Cynthia.

After fifteen years, we were part of each other's lives. But I realized, at that moment, staring at his familiar features, that I didn't really know much about his background, his life before we met.

Our conversation about the cardiac procedure had come to a sort of stalemate. Mr. Moreno decided to go forward with it, though he was unhappy about the circumstances—circumstances that I could do little to alleviate. So, to break the tension a bit, I asked him to tell me about growing up in Puerto Rico.

Without further prompting, Mr. Moreno launched into a full-fledged narrative, more voluble than I'd seen him in months. He was one of eight children, he told me. His father worked in the fields, harvesting sugarcane. One day, when he was eleven years old, he saw his father crying. He was frightened by this but gathered the courage to ask him what was wrong.

His father raised his hands in the air. "How many hands do I have?" He looked over at his son. "Two! But there are ten people in this house. My hands can't earn enough money to feed everyone."

Juan Angel (as he was called) said, "I will help you. I'll quit school and come help you in the sugarcane fields."

"No," his father said. "You have to stay in school. You have to become someone better than me."

The next day, instead of going to school, Juan Angel went to the local river and caught little fish to bring home for food. He was so proud of his contribution to the family that he begged his father to buy him his own machete in order for him to start working in the fields.

A few months short of completing fourth grade, Juan Angel joined his father in the sugarcane fields. The family's weekly income increased from thirty-five dollars to fifty-five dollars. The family was now able to eat, but Juan Angel had forever sacrificed his education.

After Juan Angel's childhood and adolescence in the scorching fields, an uncle offered to take him to Buffalo, New York, and he jumped at the chance. There, Juan Angel spent five backbreaking years on a farm, earning seventy cents an hour. He kept fifteen dollars of each week's wages and sent the rest home to Puerto Rico.

When he could tolerate fieldwork no longer, Juan Angel made his way to New York City. He hauled racks of clothes along the sidewalks of the Garment District. Then he worked as a dishwasher in a restaurant, eventually making his way up to head cook. After that, he started in the plastics factory, where he worked for twenty-seven years, quitting only at age fifty-three when he had a heart attack and ended up in my clinic at Bellevue Hospital.

Hearing even just a small part of his story put much of his life in perspective. I understood why his fiercest desire for Cynthia was that she complete school. Whenever he lamented her attitude or choice of friends or clothing, the one thing that gave him comfort was that she was still attending school every day, that she would graduate with the high-school diploma that he'd never earned. Somehow, through all the emotional chaos of Cynthia's life, some of Mr. Moreno's work ethic was seeping through.

Mr. Moreno's second cardiac procedure was, thankfully, successful and uneventful. This time when Mr. Moreno came to my clinic a few weeks after the procedure, he strode purposefully into my office, his eyes vibrant and glossy. There was no cane in sight. "I feel fantastic," he said, telling me that he'd just spent the weekend fishing in the Poconos. His weight had come down to 260—"I eat like a rabbit now," he said—and he was able to walk almost twenty blocks without fatigue.

When I listened to his heart, I was greeted with the steady metronome of a pacemaker beat. It was startling after fifteen years of listening to the jiggly rhythm of atrial fibrillation. His atria were still hiccupping along, of course, but the cardiologists had neatly severed the tie line between his atria and his ventricles, and now the ventricles contracted to the even-keeled beat of the pacemaker. This regularity afforded reliable intervals for his heart's filling and pumping, thereby allowing it to conduct oxygen to the rest of his body in a dependable manner. No wonder he felt better. And the new AICD kept to itself, withholding its powerful shocks until the moment of alarm that hopefully would never come.

As Mr. Moreno walked briskly out of my office, I thought about the many journeys he'd traveled—the one from a sugarcane plantation in Puerto Rico to Buffalo to the Lower East Side of Manhattan; the one his body had taken through the vagaries and insults of illness; the one his soul had taken with his daughter and with Cynthia. It was inspiring to see his body in its best condition ever, able to march onward.

But I could not shake off the image of the battered Juan Moreno after the first AICD debacle. That his health could swing so drastically in one direction and then another unsettled me. What might be in store for him in the next leg of his journey? This was a rock-solid man who wasn't ever going to leave his apartment, his wife, his hospital, or his doctor. We'd had fifteen years together already, and it seemed like we were going to be together for at least the next fifteen. If he was intending to cede control of all his major medical decisions to me, then I would be more than just a fellow traveler on his journey.

∞ Chapter Twenty-seven ∞

On a warm spring Monday morning, several months after Juan Moreno's second cardiac procedure, there was a frightening message on my office phone. "Your patient Dr. Chan has been admitted to the hospital."

My heart seized at hearing this. Dr. Chan was now ninety-one. To say that the physical reserve of his body was scant was generously overstating the case. Was this the beginning of the end? I wondered. Was this his biggest fear realized—that he'd die before his wife?

With dread, I tiptoed up to his hospital room, preparing myself for a heart attack, another stroke, pneumonia, diabetic complications, cancer—any one of the multitude of horrible things that could destroy this wisp of a man.

I nearly fainted with relief to learn that my fears had been wildly overblown. It was only a red swollen hand that had landed him in the hospital. It seemed that he'd had some sort of allergic reaction, but the doctors wanted to observe him overnight to be sure that it wasn't an infection. The rash was quickly treated with steroids and he was discharged the next day. I was ecstatic that it wasn't anything serious, but I soon learned that my interpretation of *serious* was different than Dr. Chan's.

When I saw him in my office two weeks after he was discharged, Dr. Chan was more agitated than I'd ever seen him. The brief course of steroids had upset his meticulously controlled blood sugar and blood pressure.

"Look at my glucose," he said, pointing to a sheet of lined paper torn from a spiral notebook. In spidery script handwriting were his daily glucose and blood-pressure values, all a bit higher than normal, but not excessively so.

I reassured him that such effects were temporary and that we'd be able to gain control of his diabetes and hypertension once the steroids wore off. I tried to convey how lucky we were that this had been such a minor illness. I thought about the setbacks Juan

Moreno, Samuel Nwanko, and Jade Collier had suffered. Their medical challenges had been far more severe, but then again they all possessed more reserve than frail Dr. Chan. Still, I tried to convince him that we had dodged the cannonballs of infirmity, that this was only a small irritation in the grand scheme of things.

Dr. Chan shook his head in a manner that conveyed disappointment more than anything else. "The balance of body...is very important," he said, gripping the paper in two tremulous hands. "Now all unbalanced. Not good."

At our next visit, several months later, Dr. Chan shuffled into my office, feet barely lifting off the ground. He brought up the allergic reaction again, concerned about its effects on his body. I reassured him that a brief course of steroids usually did not have lasting ill effects. I reminded him again that this was small potatoes compared to what could have happened. Again, he did not seem convinced. He remained quiet while I sorted through his prescriptions and lab results.

"Maybe I...go to China soon," he said, with the sort of intonation that made it unclear whether he was making a statement or asking a question.

A visit to China? I stopped what I was doing and turned to look at him. There wasn't an ounce of fat anywhere on Dr. Chan's body. He was just bones with translucent, liver-spotted skin draped over them. He sat stooped in the chair, his upper back in a permanent hunch, hands looped precariously over his cane handle. He seemed too fragile to handle the Third Avenue bus, let alone a transglobal plane ride.

"Dr. Chan," I said, "I think it's a lovely idea to visit your home, but it's fourteen hours each way on the plane. Are you sure you are up to that?"

He shrugged and handed me forms requesting an increase in hours for his wife's home attendant. I signed and stamped them.

Several weeks later, my cell phone rang while I was in the local drugstore. I'd stumbled on a two-for-one sale on zip-lock bags of all types and I figured I'd stock up. My children were rabid consumers of zip-lock bags.

I answered the phone while balancing sixteen boxes in my shopping basket. It was Dr. Chan. Something about the incongruity of talking to a patient while standing in the middle of Rite Aid wearing jeans and a tank top made me feel awkward.

"I would like...to talk to you," he said. "Where are...you now?"

I couldn't suppress the tinge of annoyance at his question. I certainly didn't want to tell him I was in the drugstore stocking up on zip-lock bags, and for the first time in our relationship I regretted giving him unfettered access. "I, uh, I'm out right now," I said as my sunglasses were dislodged by the phone.

"It is...very important," he said. "Could I...meet you...at the lobby...of your apartment building?"

Now I was truly annoyed. How presumptuous—meeting at *my* home, taking advantage of the fact that we happened to live across the street from each other. I couldn't imagine ever asking my own doctor to meet in his apartment building.

But then I saw that Dr. Chan was simply speaking to me in the only manner he knew—direct and simple. He didn't possess the linguistic skills in English for subtlety, and it wasn't fair to hold that against him. Still, I wasn't sure that I wanted to bring him to my home.

"I'll come over to your building," I said, deciding that it would be best to get whatever this was over with as soon as possible. "I think that will be easier."

Fifteen minutes later, Dr. Chan was leading me into the back garden of his apartment building where he and Mrs. Geng had pulled three lawn chairs together. Dr. Chan didn't seemed fazed as I lugged my two bulging shopping bags. I was uncomfortable to be in a doctor-patient encounter not wearing professional work clothes or a white coat.

Then it occurred to me that Dr. Chan was not a man to be put off by externals—our location, my clothes, my zeal for discounted zip-lock bags. A more acculturated American might have noticed the disconnect, might even have made a tension-defusing joke about our slightly awkward circumstances. Dr. Chan, however, didn't seem to be bothered by it, or even notice. If he didn't care, then why should I? I took off my sunglasses and relaxed my grip on the heavy shopping bags.

I sat exactly between Dr. Chan and Mrs. Geng, equidistant from both of their chairs, but I had to lean toward Dr. Chan. He was doing the talking, of course, and in order to hear his whispery voice over the New York City traffic that filtered in through the garden's gates, I had to cock my head nearly into his seat.

"I need to tell you…," he said—studiously, deliberately—"that I go to China."

I nodded my head, recalling our conversation about his going to China. I guessed he'd decided to do this vacation, and I assumed that he needed me to sign a health form for the airline.

Dr. Chan proceeded to tell me that he felt that his health had been severely jeopardized since the allergic reaction on his hand. "I need to…go back. I will…be better there. My son and daughter…care for me."

"You are going back," I said, trying to pull the story together, "to visit?"

He shook his head. "No. Back to…home."

My haze of confusion began to take a different turn. This was not a vacation—they were talking about moving back to China. I sat up and started paying closer attention. Move to China? Was this really the time in life to be relocating to the other side of the world? How would they manage the logistics? How would Mrs. Geng understand the change in locale?

But before I could ask any questions, Dr. Chan continued. "The problem, you see…is my wife not want to go," he said, gesturing toward Mrs. Geng. "She want…stay here." Mrs. Geng had three daughters living in America, and she didn't want to leave them.

"She angry that I go," Dr. Chan said. "She stay up…all night. She yell and scream. I try to…explain, but she…don't want to hear."

My head was starting to spin. "Wait a second," I said, pressing both my palms onto the arms of my chair in an attempt to right the situation. "Let me get this straight: *you* are moving to China but *she* is staying here."

Dr. Chan nodded somberly. "I invite her to come...I want her to come...but she not want to go."

Mrs. Geng couldn't follow the English, but she clearly knew what her husband was telling me, and she began to voice her objections. Despite her mental frailty, Mrs. Geng was physically far more robust than her husband, and her Mandarin boomed over his papery-thin English. I turned to look at her, then back to Dr. Chan for help with translation, then back to her as the intensity and persistence of her voice grew. I asked Dr. Chan to please translate what she was saying, but in order to hear I was forced to lean ever closer to him to make out his explanation. This seemed to be perceived by Mrs. Geng as my leaning toward his side, and so she grabbed my right arm, pulling my torso toward her. Mrs. Geng exhorted me ever more vociferously in Mandarin, seemingly physically pleading with me not to let him go to China.

I didn't know what to do. As a physician, I was supposed to advocate for my patients, but they were both my patients. For Dr. Chan, life might indeed be better in China—though I had my concerns—but his pursuing this was an obvious detriment to my patient Mrs. Geng, who was now wailing with operatic force.

I squinted my eyes and looked at Dr. Chan, unable to formulate a response. Was this the same man I'd known all these years who'd cared so scrupulously for his wife? Was this the same man who carried Mrs. Geng's purse for her, managed all her medications, cooked all her meals?

"I am...old man." Dr. Chan said. "Ninety-one years old...If I stay in America...I know I...will die. I must go...to China. My body will...be better."

Mrs. Geng's wails evolved into moans. She ran her fingers along my forearm, pressing into my muscles as though trying to milk compassion from me. Dr. Chan took my left hand in his. Both had startlingly soft skin, though Mrs. Geng's hands were fuller and fleshier than Dr. Chan's.

"B-but she is your wife," I finally stammered. "How can you leave her?"

"After a few months...," Dr. Chan said, looking down into his lap, "I think she...will forget me. That is...her disease. You know that, Doctor." He hesitated, and his voice grew even quieter. "It will likely...be better that way." There was a sadness in his demeanor that was tinged with compassion, resignation, medical knowledge, and Dr. Chan's trademark pragmatism.

Mrs. Geng was still pulling on my arm, beseeching me with a steady stream of Mandarin. I realized that Dr. Chan had not called me to ask my advice but only to inform me. My opinion was not what he was seeking. He assured me that he'd arranged a twenty-four-hour home attendant for his wife—so that was the form I'd signed for him—and that her daughters had all agreed to help care for her.

"I have...purchased ticket," he said. "My flight in...two days."

I let go of Dr. Chan and reached over to take Mrs. Geng's hand in mine, wishing I could say something—anything—to offer her some sort of comfort. Perhaps she thought I was complicit in this, that I was somehow condoning or encouraging her husband's decision.

"Please take...care of...my wife," Dr. Chan said to me. "I know you will...be good doctor to her."

There was a long and awkward pause as the discomforting finality of the situation seemed to settle on all of us. Dr Chan really was moving back to China without his wife. Mrs. Geng really was staying behind in America without her husband. What, exactly, was I supposed to say?

I stood up unsteadily, stooping to pick up two boxes of zip-lock bags that had spilled out of my shopping bags, unsure of the proper etiquette in such a situation. I asked Dr. Chan to write me a letter once he arrived in China so that I could know how he was doing and also so that I could contact him should anything happen with Mrs. Geng. I rummaged in my pockets but could not find a single scrap of paper to write on. Finally, I dug out the Rite Aid receipt from my shopping bag and wrote down my address on the back. I started to write my Bellevue address, but then I crossed it out and wrote my home address.

As I gathered up my bulging shopping bags, Dr. Chan handed me a package in a small red plastic bag as a parting gift. I thanked him, and then gave him a hug that he received awkwardly. Mrs. Geng embraced me with her solid arms, reluctant to part. I felt horribly guilty that I was somehow a party to this by not preventing her husband's departure, but I reminded myself that I was only their doctor, not their marital adviser. This was between them.

I walked gingerly across the street, grateful to return to the safety of my home to ponder what had just transpired. I flopped onto the couch, dropping my bags onto the floor. The zip-lock bags spilled out of the shopping bags, like a collapsed tower of children's blocks around my feet, burying the little red plastic bag from Dr. Chan.

How could Dr. Chan be moving back to China? Should I have tried to talk him out of it? Should I have been disgusted by his leaving his wife? Should I have been supportive of his taking initiative in his life, even at this late stage? Should I have tried to convince Mrs. Geng to move to China? Should I have argued that America was a better place for them?

I accepted that it probably was not my role to render an opinion on Dr. Chan's choice. I also accepted that Mrs. Geng had made her own choice. She still had clear enough mental faculties that this would not be considered a legal issue of abandonment. I respected that Dr. Chan had made arrangements so that his wife would be well cared for, but still...

The whole situation was unsettling. By most standards, Dr. Chan had achieved the American dream. Was it the allergic reaction that had upset everything? Or had Dr. Chan not really been happy all along, never showing it to me, or perhaps never admitting it to himself?

I thought about how his digestive system had gone awry only when he'd emigrated from China. Was this a metaphor for the downside of leaving the homeland, or was this perhaps a true damage caused by immigration? Did America slowly poison Dr. Chan until the point at which he had no choice but to abandon the promised land, even over the objections of his ill wife? How different from Julia Barquero, who felt she owed her life to America, who was convinced—probably correctly—that she would die if she returned to Guatemala.

In some ways, Dr. Chan's situation reminded me of Mohammed Ali Amal, who felt that America was a prison, despite the freedom from war and torment that it offered. Most Americans would look at Mr. Amal and think how lucky he was to have escaped Iraq and how ecstatic he should be over his good fortune in the United States. There would seem to be no rational reason to pine for return, but such emotions had no reason to be rational. The ache of displacement might simply be unimaginable to those who had never uprooted.

I stood up and in the process kicked over some of the boxes on the floor; Dr. Chan's red plastic bag lay exposed. I knelt down and opened the bag, pulling out a brand-new container of Nescafé instant coffee. Decaf. I had to smile.

Beneath the Nescafé there was a coiled leather belt tied with a bright red ribbon. An enormous golden dragon buckle dominated the belt. Last, there was a small green-and-white box of Chinese herbs. TUBER OF ELEVATED GASTRODIA, the label said, with a subtitle of HONEY AGARIC TABLETS. I turned the box over. *For arresting convulsion and tranquilizing the endopathic winds,* it read. *Effective for dizziness, infantile convulsions, epilepsy, numbed limbs, lumbago.* The rest was printed in Chinese, and there were additional handwritten Chinese instructions scribbled on top of the printed instructions.

I wondered why Dr. Chan had given me this herb. Was I supposed to prescribe this for his wife? Was this some sort of tea? Did he think I suffered from endopathic winds?

The fact that the herb was prescribed for convulsions and epilepsy concerned me, as I knew that many herbal preparations contained psychoactive compounds. Given that I had three small children with insatiable curiosities, not to mention a dog whose palate was staggeringly indiscriminate, I decided that it probably

wouldn't be wise to keep any mysterious herbs with intriguing la-
bels in the house. I tossed the box in the garbage.

I began unpacking and sorting my seeming lifetime supply of
zip-lock bags. What had I been thinking? It wasn't as though I lived
in some suburban mansion with walk-in pantries and basements
and attics for storage. I lived in a tiny Manhattan two-bedroom,
with three kids, a husband, and a seventy-five-pound black Lab.
Who was I kidding?

Of course I no longer had my receipt—that was now in Dr.
Chan's pocket—so I couldn't return anything. So instead of catching up on writing assignments, as I'd planned to, I systematically
hauled out the contents of my kitchen cabinets so that I could fit
in a quantity of plastic bags sufficient to kill off all the remaining
dolphins in the Pacific.

As I crammed the last of them in the cabinet, my eye caught that
little green-and-white box sitting on top of the garbage. My curiosity got to me. I wondered what an herb for convulsions, numbed
limbs, and endopathic winds would actually look like. What were
endopathic winds anyway? I grabbed the box and tugged open the
top. I reached in hesitantly, expecting a bag of powder. What came
out, though, was a solid object. Maybe it was some sort of ginger
root, or perhaps the indicated tuber of elevated gastrodia.

I pulled off the plastic wrapping, and instead of tubers or roots,
I discovered an intricate wooden carving. There were three spheres
within spheres, all delicately carved with flowers and dragon tails,
one inside the other. The etchings in the wood were millimeter-size,
as if carved by elves. Had the carpenter carved each part separately,
then fitted one piece inside the other? Or had it been hewn from
a solid piece of wood, with the artist masterfully carving the inner
and outer spheres simultaneously?

It came with a red braided handle for hanging, and there was,
of course, a brilliant red tail flowing from the bottom. I'd have to
visit China someday and learn if any color other than red existed
there!

The next day, I brought the carving to my office and hung it
from the corner of my bookshelf. I stared at the intricate wood-
work—the sphere within a sphere within a sphere. I was confused

about what to make of Dr. Chan and upset about the whole situation. Was Dr. Chan more manipulative and self-centered than I could have imagined? Or was he simply determined to live his life the way he needed to? How would I ever know?

I ran my finger over the whorls of the carving, feeling the infinitesimally small ridges that lined the spheres. How could so much beauty, complexity, and mystery be bound up in such a tiny object? I tried to reach my pinkie into the innermost sphere, but it was secreted away, impossible to reach. My finger was still lodged in the outer sphere when the phone rang.

"Dr. Ofri," the clerk said, "your first two patients are waiting. Also, Mr. Moya is here with a disability form, and there's a pharmacy calling for a medication refill for Juanita Tolentino. Can I transfer the call to you?"

✑ Chapter Twenty-eight ✑

I was late for the Monday-morning clinic meeting. Partly, that was because the fall weather was at its height of perfection, and I couldn't resist dallying for an extra few moments outside. Even the concrete of New York City couldn't completely mask the cidery autumnal fragrance. But the other reason I was late was the conversation I'd had with Naava and Noah that morning.

It had been more than a year since we'd returned from Costa Rica. I'd put in an immense effort at keeping Spanish alive in our home—reading Spanish stories, singing Spanish songs at night, playing up the wonders of having a "secret" language at our disposal. But I smashed up against the same cultural force that had prevented my father from passing Hebrew along to me, the same cultural force that frustrated so many immigrant parents—the impossibility of nurturing a foreign language in the all-encompassing sea of American culture. Within months of returning to New York, my kids would not speak any Spanish in response to my questions. Halfway through the school year, they didn't want to hear any stories in Spanish—even if that was the only bedtime option offered. There were plenty of Hispanic kids in their classes, but of course those kids were already fluent in English. Without having a compelling reason to speak Spanish, my children could not be induced to continue using it.

But recently, Naava had learned that a friend of hers was taking a kids' Spanish class and that there was going to be a fair amount of *helado* involved. Given the ice cream, her interest was peaked. The previous Saturday morning, after Tot Shabbat, I had taken Naava and Noah out for sushi, their favorite. After the green tea ice cream, we went to visit a Spanish class at the Instituto Cervantes. Both kids were hesitant as the teacher quizzed them to assess their level. But then he pulled out a large, globe-shaped bingo cage, and their eyes widened with awe. He let each of them spin the cage and pull out the numbers, which were to be announced in Spanish, of course. The bingo cage could be wound endlessly, like a pencil sharpener, resulting in a wonderfully raucous clatter. I stood by patiently as Naava and Noah took turns winding and winding.

This morning, Naava looked up from her cereal. "If we take that Spanish class, will we get to have sushi every Saturday?"

"Absolutely," I said. "Spanish sushi."

Noah sat up on his knees to be higher at the table. "Will there be bingo every week?" he asked, rocking his chair back and forth.

"*Creo que sí,*" I replied. "And keep that chair down. You're going to fall over backward."

Naava hesitated, not completely convinced. "Will there be green tea ice cream each week?"

"*Helado cada semana,*" I assured her.

"Will Ariel come?" Noah asked.

"No, she's too little," I said. "This would only be for the big kids."

"If we do this," said Naava, creating deliberative circles in her cereal with her spoon that seemed to coincide with the machinations of her mind, "then we'll have Hebrew in the morning, Japanese for lunch, and Spanish in the afternoon."

"*Exactamente,*" I said, and didn't feel it necessary to say that the sushi restaurant was run entirely by Malaysians.

"Okay," she said slowly. "I think I'll try it."

As I walked to work that morning, I felt exhilarated by the autumn air, and exhilarated by my children's willingness to try a Spanish class, even if it was entirely based on a bingo cage and green tea ice cream. Maybe I'd actually done something right as a parent. Maybe all that effort to live in Costa Rica for a year would actually offer them that second language. Maybe they'd thank me someday for giving them that opportunity.

I walked briskly through the waiting room, trying to get to the conference room without being too late for the meeting. As I passed by the rows of chairs, I spotted Julia Barquero and gave a quick wave. She did not have an appointment with me; she was seeing the nurse to have her Coumadin level checked, and I passed by quickly. My hand was on the conference room door when something made me turn back and look again. Julia seemed different today, somehow smaller and more contracted into her space. Her shoulders slumped from her neck as though they were weighted. Her face had a wan expression that I'd never seen before.

"*¿Está bien?*" I asked, walking back toward her. "Is it Vasco?" She shook her head no. Vasco was fine—he was now living with her and Lucita. "For the past month," she said, "it's like I'm swimming through mud. I can hardly take a step."

Her description frightened me. Julia had never lacked for energy. She'd always been able to climb the three flights of stairs to her apartment. I decided to skip my meeting.

I listened to Julia's heart and lungs. I was relieved to see that there were no clinical signs of congestive heart failure—edematous legs or wet lungs. But something was clearly wrong. There was nothing I could find to suggest an infection or other cause for her weakness. I began to get nervous that it was her heart.

What if we'd finally reached that precipice that I'd feared? What if the actin and myosin fibers of Julia's heart had reached the limits of their malleability? What if we'd exhausted the regenerative munificence of her young body? If what we were seeing was the end of Julia's ability to compensate for a failing heart, then there would be nothing to do but watch her slide toward death.

I called her cardiologist. He hoped that maybe it was a failing valve—a valve, at least, could be replaced. We arranged for Julia to see him tomorrow. The next day I left for a trip to California to give a lecture. On the five-hour flight I thought about Julia. We'd talked about this book I was writing and she'd readily agreed to let me write about her. I'd already made a lot of progress on the chapter about her, but it wasn't finished. I'd intended to close it with a meditation about the quandary of transplantation for undocumented immigrants. But it could remain a semitheoretical issue, a parlor debate...as long as Julia remained clinically stable.

When I'd first met Julia, we simply accepted it as fact that it was impossible for her to get onto the transplant list. But when I started writing about her, nearly a year ago, it was the first time I'd ever stopped to really consider the specifics of this dilemma. I contacted the United Network for Organ Sharing, the umbrella organization that coordinated the various U.S. transplant centers. I learned that

American citizens received 96 percent of the organs; legal residents (immigrants with green cards) received 3 percent. The remaining 1 percent of organs went to foreigners, but there was no information as to whether these foreigners were visitors from other countries or illegal immigrants living in the United States. (Interestingly, foreigners *donated* 2 percent of all organs.)

Armed with that information, I'd called Julia's cardiologist and asked if the cardiology team could revisit the transplant issue. There was a slim chance—1 percent, maybe—that Julia might be able to get on the list.

"I'll go back over her records," the cardiologist had said at that time. "But the truth is, she can't get on the list right now anyway, because her functional status is excellent. It will only come into play when she gets sicker."

Now, as I wrote about Julia's abruptly worsening condition one year later, I worried whether we'd reached that point. Gazing out the window of the airplane, I watched the endless Midwest plains go by, followed by the snow-covered Rockies. I was startled anew by how vast the country was. Somewhere to my left was the Mexican border, and somewhere along those two thousand miles was the spot where Julia Barquero had walked from a fate of certain death to a fate of near-certain death.

Forty-eight hours later, as soon as I arrived home from California, I paged the cardiologist. While I dialed the phone, I pulled up Julia's medical record in the computer. Even before he called back, I saw that she'd been admitted to the hospital. As the phone rang, I could see that she'd been transferred from the regular ward to the ICU. This couldn't be good.

The cardiologist confirmed what I had feared: it was her heart muscle that was failing, not a valve. It was a testament to Julia's strong body that she still did not have significant fluid backed up in her lungs and legs, but the arterial pressure in her lungs had skyrocketed, confirming that her ventricles were buckling. The inpatient doctors had given her diuretics to try to ease this pressure, but then her blood pressure bottomed out. Now they'd moved her to the ICU. Here they could infuse pressors to bolster her blood pressure to allow some wiggle room for the diuretics. This fragile arrangement worked, and she was feeling a bit better. The catch was, however, that pressors could only be given intravenously in an ICU. She couldn't leave the hospital until either her ventricular function improved slightly or a heart transplant became available. Otherwise she'd have to live her remaining days in the ICU, tethered to an IV pole.

"I did my residency at Columbia," the cardiology fellow said. "I know the transplant people there and I'll present her case. Let's see if we can get them to take her."

"What happens if they don't?" I asked.

"We'll talk to the folks at Mount Sinai. They have a smaller program, but they're worth a shot."

"What happens if they don't take her?"

"Well, we'll try at Montefiore."

"And if that doesn't work?"

He was silent.

✍ Chapter Twenty-nine ✍

It wasn't even clear why she'd been admitted to Bellevue. It was one of those bleak, frigid days in the lingering tail of December. Night fell by midafternoon, it seemed, and daytime offered only the scrawniest threads of sunlight. Her husband and son lived in China. She indicated that she had no family here in America. Now she was sitting in a room on Seventeen West, and the team and I were struggling with the Mandarin interpreter on the telephone to figure out why Xui-Ping Liang was here.

Slim, youthful-appearing, with sleek black hair gathered in a high ponytail, Mrs. Liang sat up in the bed with the phone crammed against her ear, chattering rapidly with the interpreter. She gestured animatedly to make her points, but we couldn't tell which among her words she was emphasizing.

The story came through that she'd been called about an abnormal lab value and was told to come to the hospital. But in scanning the labs in the computer, we couldn't find anything grossly amiss. There was a clinic visit yesterday during which her doctor tested her thyroid level. The results came back mildly elevated, and the doctor had called her later that day, reminding her to take her thyroid pills, commenting in his note about the patient's noncompliance with her thyroid treatment. Perhaps Mrs. Liang had misunderstood the message and thought she had to come to the ER. Once in the ER, she somehow managed to get herself admitted to the hospital—and we couldn't figure out why. She couldn't offer any sort of chief complaint or anything that was bothering her.

Mrs. Liang certainly had enough illnesses under her belt, though that alone shouldn't have been cause for admission. At the age of fifty-one she'd already been through breast cancer and now had colon cancer raging through her body. Despite a year of aggressive chemotherapy, the colon cancer had spread to her liver, spine, and lungs. But she didn't look nearly as ill as her medical record suggested. Her unwrinkled face looked two decades younger than her stated age, and with the sheet pulled up, you could barely see the bulge of her cancerous abdomen on her otherwise slender frame.

When pressed, Mrs. Liang said she had a little pain in her belly but generally felt well. She told us that she lived alone and despite her illness had no trouble getting to and from her second-floor walk-up, doing her own shopping and cooking. She didn't seem that sick to us—why had the ER docs admitted her to the hospital? Had they seen something we didn't? Had their interpreter uncovered some symptom that we were not able to elicit?

Though her appetite wasn't what it used to be, Mrs. Liang had—as the oncologists put it—excellent performance status. Performance status was considered to be the best predictor of outcome, no matter what the stage of the disease. Mrs. Liang was up and about, with full energy—not bed-bound, stricken, consumed by disease. Which seemed startling to us when we reviewed the CT scan of her abdomen.

Mrs. Liang's liver was massively enlarged, watermelon-size—easily the largest liver I'd ever seen in my life. It was jam-packed with metastatic lesions, like a bulbous basket crammed with tennis balls. Radiologists are normally meticulous about the number and dimensions of lesions, down to the millimeter size, but in this case the report simply stated that the lesions were "too numerous to count."

When we reviewed the CT of her chest, there was that phrase again—"too numerous to count"—this time referring to the metastatic lesions in her lungs. Here, the lungs resembled baskets crammed with Ping-Pong balls.

The resilience and reserve of the liver are legendary, and Mrs. Liang was robustly demonstrating that clinical pearl. Despite the fact that almost every centimeter of her hepatic tissue had been invaded by tumor, the blood tests of liver function were nearly normal. Whatever liver was left was working just fine, producing adequate amounts of necessary proteins. Her liver enzymes, which start to climb during liver damage, were only modestly elevated, in the 200s.

Similarly, despite the cancer's near-total invasion of her lungs, Mrs. Liang was breathing comfortably. She must have descended from sturdy stock, because whatever viable lung and liver tissue remained was functioning remarkably well, keeping her body at a near-normal performance status.

The resident and interns reviewed the CT scan with me. The word used in medicine for a scan like that was *impressive*. An outsider might think the doctors were being callous, looking only at the disease and not the person. But the word was used with a sense of being unnerved by the potent biology of cancer, of being humbled and awed by a pathology of such force. It *was* an impressive scan.

But what floored us more was when Mrs. Liang asked us—via the translator—what we would be doing to cure her disease.

Cure her disease?

Did she not know what her scans showed? Did she not understand about the relentless spread of the disease?

Cure?

Maybe, like Mr. Ptchetpchdad, she'd been told but didn't understand. Or maybe she understood but was in denial. Or maybe the information hadn't quite traversed the translation channels accurately. Perhaps, as Evans had told me about Haiti, her culture had no concept of a disease like cancer. Maybe, like Nazma Uddin, she had unrealistic expectations about what American medicine could do for her. Maybe, like Juan Moreno, she'd had a bad experience with the medical system. Or maybe she simply did not know about her diagnosis; perhaps her doctors, like Julia Barquero's, were too afraid to say. The permutations of confusion and misunderstanding were endless.

In the best of circumstances, such conversations were difficult—delivering horrible news, piercing layers of denial, bringing blunt truths to the forefront—and we relied on our abilities to speak empathically, sometimes metaphorically. We used verbal language, body language, eye contact to form connections. We gauged the ability to press forward by the patient's responses, both subtle and obvious.

With someone like Juan Moreno, who spoke English fluently, I could rely on my instincts in navigating a difficult conversation. With Señoras Ortiz and Estrella, I had the language skills for ordinary conversation, but when things grew complicated or emotional, my lack of sophistication in Spanish became a handicap. Mrs. Geng could only communicate her protests to me via her husband, who was the cause of her angst and could not have been an objective interpreter.

With Julia Barquero, her grim prognosis was told to her with the necessity of a translator phone. Similarly, with Mr. Ptchetpchdad, we had to discuss his most painful memory via a telephone interpreter. Most of my Monday SOT patients had to reveal the torture they'd experienced through a telephone service. To me, inserting a telephone as a go-between in such delicate processes was like adding construction boots to a pas de deux.

We did our best to explain everything to Mrs. Liang—the cancer, the metastases—as honestly and gently as possible as the cycles of translation looped back and forth across the telephone wires, but it felt awkward and disjointed. What sort of tone was the interpreter using with Mrs. Liang? Did he sound empathetic to her? Businesslike? Bored? We couldn't tell. And what sort of tone was Mrs. Liang using in reply? Did she seem confused? Surprised? Upset? Numb?

We were elated when we learned that her regular oncologist spoke Mandarin. This would clear up all the misunderstandings— a doctor she was familiar with, in the appropriate specialty, who spoke her language, who could explain directly what was happening.

Several hours were spent paging, calling, tracking down this holy grail of the Mandarin-speaking oncologist. These hours were ultimately fruitless, as we finally pieced together that that the oncologist was on vacation and not due to return until after New Year's. Luckily, New Year's was only four days away. We decided that the hard discussion about the big picture could probably wait until Mrs. Liang's oncologist got back. We'd just focus on stabilizing the current issues for the moment.

Except that we didn't know what those current issues were, because Mrs. Liang seemed to be feeling pretty well, with no specific complaints. No one knew how it was that she came to be admitted to the hospital, but it was already nighttime on an icy December evening. We decided that we'd just let her rest for the night and try to sort things out in the morning, maybe even discharge her if she had no real need to be in the hospital.

But the next day Mrs. Liang felt slightly worse. She pointed to her belly, and we palpated it. It was maybe a touch more distended, perhaps a tad firmer, a little more tender. The bowel sounds seemed maybe a few degrees quieter than yesterday. The morning labs showed that her liver enzymes had climbed a little, from the 200s to the 300s. An X-ray showed that her liver was pressing on her intestine, preventing stool and gas from passing—a partial small-bowel obstruction. With a liver that size, a partial small-bowel obstruction wasn't unexpected; it had probably occurred on and off over the past year. Luckily, it was easy to treat by the insertion of a simple nasogastric tube to relieve the pressure.

Perhaps it was a good thing, in the end, that she was in the hospital—whatever reason had brought her here—so that this obstruction could be treated in its earliest stages. We still didn't know why she'd been admitted, but at least we now had something to treat.

The intern slid a nasogastric tube through Mrs. Liang's nose and down to her stomach, and then attached it to suction so that it would remove the accumulated gas and liquid. Mrs. Liang bristled at the uncomfortable sensation of the tube in her nose, and fiddled with it constantly, but by the next morning she reported feeling better—softer belly, normal bowel sounds. She seemed back to her baseline.

Her blood tests, however, told a different story. Her liver enzymes had now tripled to more than 1,000, her white blood cell count had gone up, and she had an elevated lactate level. An elevated lactate was a nonspecific sign that tissues somewhere in the body were not getting enough oxygen. It could result from severe infection, congestive heart failure, respiratory failure, liver failure, renal failure, toxic ingestion—any one of a host of biologic mayhems. The only guaranteed aspect of an elevated lactate was that it wasn't good news.

The small-bowel obstruction could have potentially explained all the abnormal blood tests—except for that fact that Mrs. Liang was clinically improved with the nasogastric tube in place.

Something else calamitous might be brewing. Mrs. Liang could have an infection somewhere. She could have intrinsic liver failure, the cancer having finally overwhelmed the organ. She could have been experiencing kidney failure that resulted from liver failure—the poorly understood but uniformly disastrous hepatorenal syndrome. Or she could have all of the above.

With extensive cancer in so many organs, Mrs. Liang was a setup for a myriad of pathological processes. *But the most concerning issue*, I wrote in my progress note that day, *is that the patient does not seem aware of the severity of illness.* We started broad-spectrum antibiotics and IV fluids, hoping to treat whatever might be treatable.

It turned out that her oncologist was actually away for two weeks, and wouldn't be returning to the hospital any time soon. We'd have to address the big picture—particularly the issue of advance directives—right now. The elevated lactate and worsening liver enzymes compelled us to do so.

We sat with the translator on the phone, trying to explain lactates and liver enzymes. We attempted to discuss the delicate issues of CPR, resuscitation, ICU. But Mrs. Liang kept talking about curing the disease. She said she wanted everything done.

It was clear to me that there were some enormous misunderstandings going on and that we'd need the help of someone who knew her, someone who could bridge both cultures and both languages.

"Do you have anyone who could help us talk together about what's going on?" the resident asked via the translator.

"I have two brothers and one sister," Mrs. Liang replied.

"I know you have family in China," he said, "but do you have anyone here in America? It doesn't have to be family—it could be close friends."

"My brothers live in Queens," Mrs. Liang said.

Queens? She had family here in New York? She'd never told us that.

The resident pressed her some more, but it turned out that none of her siblings spoke English. But maybe there was a nephew or a niece who did. Was there a phone number? Could we call?

Mrs. Liang started reciting a phone number. As the resident obtained the digits from the interpreter, he announced them out loud, and I scribbled them hurriedly on the back of an EKG.

I quickly dialed this new number, hoping for a lead, someone close to Mrs. Liang, someone who spoke English. Ideally a niece or nephew who wasn't a minor. The phone rang and I anxiously awaited the pickup, potentially the key to communication with Mrs. Liang. The phone rang in my ear, and then there was a strange parallel buzzing within the room. It rang again in my ear, and again came the buzzing. Something vibrated on the nightstand. Mrs. Liang's own cell phone. She had given us her own phone number.

The following day, Mrs. Liang's enzymes doubled to 2,500. She was sleepier, and her blood pressure was a bit lower, but she answered our questions. We were able to extract another phone number from her—another niece or nephew—but no one answered when I called. I left a message to please call as soon as possible.

That night was New Year's Eve. Before we left for the evening, the team and I reviewed her case. We considered all the possible reversible issues of her worsening liver enzymes—infection, dehydration, bowel obstruction. All of these were being treated. If her liver function was declining because of any of these, there could be a chance of improvement. If, however, the liver was declining because of the overwhelming cancer, there really wasn't any other option beyond palliative care.

That night, Mrs. Liang's blood pressure dropped even lower. The overnight team was nervous and called the medical consult (the senior medical resident on duty). The medical consult felt that Mrs. Liang should be moved immediately to the ICU, that she needed blood tests every four hours to follow her critical condition. She wrote in her note that because the patient specifically stated "she wanted everything done," the doctors were "ethically obligated" to begin intensive therapy to raise her blood pressure.

I was livid the next morning when I read those words in the chart. Two new medical students had materialized on our team that day—new ones were scheduled to come at the beginning of each month—and they shuffled their feet awkwardly as I ranted about the heinous misjudgment of the medical consult.

No bed had been available in the ICU overnight, so Mrs. Liang had been moved to the observation unit, a step below the ICU.

An oxygen mask obscured her face. The resident and I asked her questions, but she was unable to answer. We held the translator phone to her ear, hoping the sound of Mandarin would perk her up, but she just mumbled, and her head sagged away from us like a top-heavy squash lolling on its vine. Her skin was sallow, her lips now parched. Her hair hung in dull clumps, and her eyes remained closed with chalky debris accumulating in the corners. She resisted our touch, seeming uncomfortable in every position. The transformation over four days was frightening. From a walking, talking person, Mrs. Liang had turned into a limp, stuporous body.

Xui-Ping Liang was now actively dying.

It wasn't often that we were witnesses to the exact turning point in a disease, but in this case we were—thanks, perhaps, to a prescient ER physician. From the time cancer had first taken root in Mrs. Liang's colon many years ago, her body had compensated with impressive efficiency. Like Julia Barquero's, Mrs. Liang's hardy constitution protected her from the clinical consequences of the spreading disease. It kept her lungs functioning; it kept her liver working; it kept her mind intact; it allowed her to walk, cook, eat, converse—it allowed her to live an essentially normal life.

The day that Mrs. Liang was admitted to Bellevue marked the final day of this remarkable physiologic compensation. Overnight, she reached the tipping point, and, like Julia's, her body was no longer able to withstand the onslaught. And when the waters breached the levees, every organ system was taken down in its wake—liver, kidneys, vascular system, nervous system, lungs. It wasn't a matter of simply treating the possible reversible causes—which of course we were doing—it was that the entire body was failing, disintegrating within a week before our very eyes.

"The medical consult wrote incorrectly in the chart," I explained to the medical students. "There is no 'ethical obligation' to provide care that is not medically indicated. A liver transplant or a lung transplant would seem preposterous in a situation like this, and we would never think to offer it. ICU care should be thought of in the same way," I said, pounding my fist on the chart for emphasis, "only to be considered when it is medically appropriate. ICU care is only meant to be a bridge, a support while the underlying disease is treated."

We stood silently, gazing at Mrs. Liang, who seemed to have shrunk to half her size in the few days that we'd known her. "Mrs. Liang's underlying disease," I said, curling my arms around the chart, hugging it toward my chest, "cannot be treated."

The intern spent the entire day working the phones. He finally tracked down a nephew, who then got the sister. The sister called a brother. His daughter got the other brother. After hours of phone tag and relays and messages, we were able to communicate that they all needed to come to the hospital as soon as possible for a family meeting.

By 3:00 p.m., three siblings and four nieces and nephews had assembled in the hallway. The resident brushed the bagel crumbs off the table in the conference room as we ushered the family in. The three siblings appeared much older than Mrs. Liang. Their faces were wrinkled, tired. They dressed simply and practically, in utilitarian dun-colored clothing. Their children, who all appeared to be in their twenties and early thirties, dressed sharply—far more fashionably than any of the medical team gathered at the table— with trendy haircuts and designer handbags and eyeglasses.

It was only Sun-Yee, though, the twenty-four-year-old niece with an oval face and rimless glasses, who could speak fluent English. I offered the family the opportunity to bring in a hospital interpreter or to use the translator phone, but they all indicated that they preferred Sun-Yee to translate.

I asked them what they understood of Mrs. Liang's illness. The siblings spoke through Sun-Yee and told us that Mrs. Liang had indeed told them that she had colon cancer, but she'd never mentioned that it had spread to other parts of her body. This was the first they were learning of it.

They were shocked to see her in this condition—almost un-arousable, moaning, not responding to them. When they'd seen her before New Year's she'd been alert and communicative.

I explained the situation as clearly and as honestly as I could. I was acutely aware that my resident and interns were watching me, and that not only did I need to do the right thing for the patient, I also needed to model the right thing for my team. And of course there was the new crop of medical students. This was their first day on the medical ward.

As a rule, I tried to lay out all possibilities for a patient and family, offering as much choice as is possible. The simplest approach, the one I'd seen countless doctors take, was to say: "Would you like us to do everything or would you like us to let nature take its course?"

On the surface, the appeal of this approach for the doctor was that it fulfilled the dictates of patient autonomy. On a deeper level, I think that doctors were drawn to this approach because it allowed us to avoid the emotional cost of taking a stand.

Doing everything versus *letting nature take its course* was a false choice when someone was dying of liver failure from metastatic cancer. I'm sure that the medical consult was aware of that on New Year's Eve. She knew the dismal medical facts as well as anyone. She knew that all the ICU care in the world would not change the precipitous fury of Mrs. Liang's cancer. Whether she was fearful of lawsuits or simply not confident in her own medical judgment, she'd dodged the issue under the guise of patient autonomy. The fact that the patient had voiced the words "I want everything done" allowed the medical consult to avoid the difficult decision.

Earlier in my career, I probably would have done the same thing. Better to err on the side of doing something than doing nothing. Better to err on the side of patient autonomy than medical paternalism.

But I felt different now. What I'd once viewed as medical bravery—rushing a dying patient to the ICU, unleashing the full gamut of medical technology—now smacked of cowardice.

Presenting such a choice bordered on political theater. The two choices—*doing everything* or *letting nature take its course*—were not at all equal. The real choices—and the medical consult knew this—were dying in the ICU on a ventilator with round-the-clock medical monitoring or dying in a regular room without these accoutrements. Death was going to be present in either option. The only difference was style.

Using Sun-Yee as the interpreter, I explained that Mrs. Liang was dying of liver failure related to her cancer. I told the family that the cancer was not curable and that it was affecting her kidneys, lungs, and brain. I told them that options in the ICU might extend her life by a few days, but that it would not change the inevitability of her death.

They all sat quietly as Sun-Yee translated my words for the older generation.

I looked around at my team—resident, two interns, two medical students—and then turned back to the family. "In my opinion, I do not think it would be wise to send Mrs. Liang to the ICU," I said. "It would not ultimately help her, and might cause her more discomfort. I recommend that we start a morphine drip to control her pain. This could possibly hasten her death, but I think she will be more comfortable this way."

I listened to myself speak. For a moment I felt a flash of old-fashioned paternalism. Was I unduly pressuring the family? Was I being overbearing, insisting on my own philosophy of end-of-life care?

I explained to the family about a DNR, and why I felt that resuscitation would offer more discomfort than benefit. For each of the concepts I introduced, I stopped and solicited their opinions. With the niece translating, this took a long time, but it gave us the opportunity to observe their faces and body language. Over the course of the conversation, there was a subtle but unmistakable relaxation.

The family felt that Mrs. Liang, despite what she'd verbalized, would prefer a quieter death, even if it came somewhat sooner, to a prolonged ICU death. What the family was most anxious about was that Mrs. Liang's body be sent back to her husband and son in China for burial. I confessed that I didn't know anything about international body transfers. Something else to learn.

Within thirty minutes we had moved Mrs. Liang from the observation unit to a private room and started the morphine drip. It took only a low dose for her moaning and writhing to immediately stop. We switched the oxygen face mask to a less obtrusive nasal-cannula tube that sat just below her nostrils so the family could see her face. We gave the family twenty-four-hour visiting passes and instructed the front desk to allow as many visitors for as long as they wanted.

When we arrived the next morning for rounds, Mrs. Liang was already dead. She'd died at 2:30 a.m., less than twelve hours after our family conversation. The night nurse said there was no evidence of distress.

Two weeks after Mrs. Liang died, my month on the wards ended. Too tired to sort out my accumulated papers and equipment at work, I'd hauled everything home and was going through them on my living room floor. I made piles of the loose papers, separating ones that I needed to file, ones that contained some issue to follow up on, ones that needed to be shredded for confidentiality, and ones that I couldn't decide about. I rifled through the pockets of my white coat and pulled out my pens, stethoscope, prescription pad, and ink stamper—all the equipment I'd been using for the month. I balled the dirty coat into a plastic bag, annoyed that I'd forgotten, yet again, to drop it off at the hospital laundry. In the middle of the papers, I stumbled across a scrap of paper with the phone number of Mrs. Liang's niece.

So often we mean to contact a family after a death but never do, as more patients and more clinical clutter fill our brains. This time around, my disorganization had given me the chance. I dialed Sun-Yee's number.

"I guess we're doing okay," Sun-Yee said in response to my question, exhaling deeply. "Better than before. The hardest part was arranging to get my aunt's body sent back to China. Now that it is finally on its way, everybody can rest easy."

"I'm sorry that I didn't have a chance to get to know your aunt very well while she was alive," I said. I paused, staring at the piles of papers on the floor that seemed so oppressive at that moment. "Could you...would you mind telling me a little bit about her?"

Sun-Yee's voice perked up immediately. "My aunt was such a happy person. She had lots of friends in China. She went to church regularly and sang in the choir."

"How did she come to America?" I asked.

"It was just a vacation," Sun-Yee explained. "She came for a visit, five years ago, to see her siblings in America. She came by herself because her husband was working and her son was in school. She had vacation from her job, so she came here for a few weeks. But then she got sick."

A vacation? I closed my eyes for a moment, thinking about the vacations I'd taken in my life, contemplating how Mrs. Liang's had been so harshly disrupted.

"Why didn't she go home at that point?" I asked.

"She wanted to," Sun-Yee said, "but she felt that she could get better medical treatment in America. She trusted Western medicine more than Eastern medicine. Her husband and son wanted to visit her, but they weren't able."

An image of Dr. Chan came to my mind at that moment. He'd felt the exact opposite—that his body could only heal if he returned to his homeland in China.

"When your aunt first came to the hospital," I said to Sun-Yee, "she told us that her only family was in China, that she had no family in America. But all her siblings live here. Why do you think she said that?"

"She was a very strong woman," Sun-Yee said. "She took care of everything herself, and never wanted to depend on anyone. She was the type of person who kept bad things inside. She told you that she didn't have any family in America because she didn't want us to be troubled by her problems. She didn't want us to know how sick she was."

"Do you think *she* understood how sick she was?"

Sun-Yee was silent for a moment. "I can't answer that," she said awkwardly. "But she was a nurse in China. She knew a lot about the body."

After we hung up the phone, I grabbed the piles of papers from the floor and shoved them back in my bag—I'd deal with them another time. I took out my cello and tightened the hairs on the bow. Klengel's Concertino in C was opened on the stand, dog-eared and strewn with pencil marks from six months of work. Six months and I'd only now been able to turn to page three.

Twelve measures of triplets faced me—forty-eight consecutive triplets that lilted over exacting half tones. Such chromatic half tones were a piece of cake on the piano, an inconsequential stroll from the black keys to the white keys. On a stringed instrument, however, these half tones had no demarcation other than the painstaking distinction by one's own ear.

I started down the line of triplets, straining my ears to snag the correct intervals between notes, shifting my fingers in ever more minute adjustments. Mrs. Liang—a nurse. How could that be? It was one thing for a layperson to be confused about cancer, but quite another thing for a medical professional.

Over and over I plowed through the lines, wincing at the obvious imperfections. How I longed for perfect pitch, to know with absolute certainty that an F-sharp was an F-sharp. I'd be grateful even for relative pitch, to know for sure that the interval from the A string to the D string was a perfect fifth. I'd be able to tune my instrument by ear, like any respectable cellist, rather than by sneaking furtive glances at my electronic tuner.

A nurse? How could a nurse have been asking about cure while in the throes of widely metastatic disease? Could she have been in that much denial?

I started again from the top of the page, up and down the chromatic steps. Half tones, whole tones, double-flats—how could I ever make my ear hear these correctly? And then there were the mechanics of the bow: The first twenty-four sets of triplets used a single bow stroke for each three notes. The next six broke up the bowing within the triplet. The next eight were completely different —unbalanced and alternating. Periodically, I had to stop and give my brain a rest lest it sputter to a halt like an engine overgunned.

But Mrs. Liang wasn't just any nurse. She was a nurse who had left her husband and son for a vacation and found herself stranded eight thousand miles away, mired in illness for five long years. I wished I could have known her for some of that time so that she wouldn't have had strangers attending her at the very end of her life.

Maybe the only thing driving her forward during those five years was the need to get back to China to see her family. Perhaps the only way she could live each of those eighteen hundred days was to focus on her illness being cured, because cure meant home. Her denial may have served a critical purpose.

Back again through the triplets. Up and down the fingerboard trying to keep track of the alternating bow direction along with the half-tone intonations. Some measures were marked *piano*, others *forte*. There were crescendos and decrescendos to pay attention to.

I was exhausted just contemplating all these variables, tempted to slam the book closed. But I couldn't. Once I'd played the music a few times, the chromatic dissonance began to melt, and the haunting harmonies became apparent. Once I'd gained enough facility to plow through the lines without stopping, hints of beauty rose to the surface. The intricate melody began to take shape and it pulled me in. Even if I could never perfect it, the longing had been kindled and there was nothing else I could do but persevere.

I imagined the plane landing in the Beijing airport. Maybe her husband and son—now a young man—would be permitted onto the tarmac. A simple pine coffin would be unloaded and the two of them in matching white shirts would step forward to assist the baggage handlers. Brushing off the admonitions of the handlers, they'd each grab a corner of the coffin, easing it onto the waiting cart. They'd walk alongside the cart, flanking each side of the coffin, eyes focused straight ahead, hands firmly cupping the wooden box—a still life of wordless focus within the noisy airport bustle—guiding Xui-Ping Liang home.

Although there would be a funeral in the church, they would first bring Mrs. Liang to their home. Their house would have already been prepared. The mirrors would have been taken down and there would be a white cloth draping the door. Incense and candles would sit on the family altar, next to a photo of Mrs. Liang from before she left China. A plate of food would be waiting to be placed by the coffin as a traditional offering.

When Mrs. Liang left for her vacation but didn't come back, her husband probably did not touch her things. As the years passed, her possessions might have gathered into a progressively smaller and smaller corner of the house, but they were never removed. It would be easy, then, for Mr. Liang to retrieve one of her combs now, as it would have remained on the far shelf in the bathroom.

The coffin would be balanced on two low wooden stools, with the head directed toward the inside of the home. Mr. Liang would snap the comb in half, as was tradition. Only then would he and his son combine the effort of their four hands to raise the lid of the coffin.

The lid would creak at first; then it would open silently. The faint smell of sawdust and of jasmine would rise from the box. Mrs. Liang's body—embalmed and prepared half a world away in Chinatown, New York—would lie before them. Her face would be covered with a yellow square of silk, her body draped with a long blue cloth. The contours of her body would be visible. Husband and son would stare downward only, not at each other.

Mr. Liang's hand hesitates before the yellow covering, unable to lift it. But his son edges in and reaches his own lean hand under his father's wrinkled one. He hasn't seen his mother since he was a boy and knows only the photograph that hangs on the wall. Gently easing the cloth from beneath his father's hand, he tugs it free. His mother's face appears smaller than he remembers, as though she has been miniaturized. It isn't her, but it is.

Mr. Liang slips one half of the broken comb on the satin pillow, next to his wife's smooth dark hair. The other half he grips in his hand, feeling the teeth needle into his skin. This half will be placed on the family altar, but not just yet. The son gives the yellow cloth a gentle shake to smooth out the creases. He pauses for a moment, unblinking, to be sure he memorizes what he sees, then he carefully lays the silk cloth back over his mother's face, making certain the broken comb is included under the covering. Mrs. Liang has finally come home.

∾ Chapter Thirty ∾

Despite all the talk of global warming, the first week in March managed to bring a full-fledged northeaster. Ten inches of snow were dumped on the streets of Manhattan on a Sunday night, prompting the first snow day of the New York City public schools in five years. Noah insisted on holding the leash when we walked Juliet that morning, and both boy and dog rippled with excitement, hurling their bodies into the pristine snowdrifts with abandon. Frankly, I was equally tempted to plunge into the snow and spend the day in the enticing whiteness. But I figured that I needed to show up to work since I was likely one of the few physicians who could. Most of my colleagues were probably still shoveling out their driveways in the distant suburbs, and I had the mixed blessing of living within walking distance of Bellevue.

I figured it would be a slow day at clinic, as was typically the case on bad-weather days, but amazingly, every patient showed up. The waiting room looked straight out of North Dakota—people in thick puffy coats, industrial boots, gargantuan wool hats, mufflers wound up to their eyes, trails of wet snow snaking along the floor.

But the biggest miracle was Julia Barquero, sitting in my office, wearing an oversize pink sweater, smiling casually at me as though beating death at its own game hadn't been a big deal. It had taken weeks in the ICU, but gradually her heart muscle recovered enough to wean off the intravenous pressors. Maybe it had just been a viral infection that had pushed her over the edge—we'd never know for sure—but somehow she'd managed to claw her way back to her baseline. Of course, her baseline was still a poorly pumping heart that would never improve to normal.

Once again, to look at Julia, you'd never know. She could again climb the three flights of stairs to her apartment, she could take Vasco and Lucita to school, she could make it to her doctor's appointment in the middle of an urban blizzard. You wouldn't know. But I knew.

"It feels so good to feel good again," she said in Spanish, and a flush rose in her cheeks, as though she were embarrassed to admit this.

"And it feels so good to see you this way," I replied, but immediately wanted to swallow back the words. It did feel good, but it also felt awful. We'd won this round, but we were still doomed to lose. Julia Barquero's life was still a chronicle of a death foretold, and this bitter fact soured the joy I might have had about her current remission.

"*¿Y sus hijos?*" she asked, pointing to the picture on my desk of Naava, Noah, and Ariel. "*¿Cómo están sus hijos?*"

I was relieved that she shifted the topic of conversation. I told her that Naava and Noah had been taking a Saturday-afternoon Spanish class, and I was hoping that it would keep their Spanish alive in their brains. But I really needed to bring them to a Spanish-speaking country again.

"*Guatemala es un país hermoso a visitar,*" Julia said.

"I know," I said, and I told her how I'd once visited Guatemala with a fellow intern. It was the first time I'd ever taken a Spanish class abroad.

"*¿Lo gozó?*" she asked, eyebrows raised expectantly as though she were suddenly the official representative of her country.

"*¡Sí, mucho!*" I replied. I'd enjoyed the trip immensely. I told her about visiting the small Mayan villages surrounding the wondrous Lake Atitlán, shadowed by a trio of blue-gray volcanoes. About the time we'd spent in the touristy but still beautiful highland towns of Antigua, Quetzaltenango, Panajachel, and Chichicastenango, but that the highlight of the trip was Tikal.

At the mention of these famous Mayan ruins, Julia let out a meditative sigh. "Ubalo and I had planned to visit Tikal for our honeymoon," she said in Spanish, "but it didn't work out. Then Vasco was born, then he got sick, so we never went." Her eyes cut a wistful arc across the room, as though imagining the trip that never was.

"It was truly memorable," I said. "One of the highlights of my life."

"Could you..." Julia hesitated. "Could you tell me about it?"

I leaned forward on my desk, pressing my forearms onto the

litter of papers, trying to conjure up that trip. The first week of Spanish classes—four hours a day, one-on-one—plus living with a family gave me a boost of confidence to spend the next week traveling with my basic Spanish phrases. Tikal was located in the far northeastern reaches of the country, in a dense, humid rain forest of towering ceiba trees, tropical cedars, and mahogany. For centuries, this enormous pre-Columbian city had been buried in the jungle, and even now it was nearly impossible to reach over land. We flew in a rickety plane that shuddered rhythmically with the winds.

I described to Julia the pyramidal temples in the center of the site, each two hundred feet tall. Climbing the steps gave me vertigo, but we persevered. From the summit there was an undisturbed view of miles of jungle. With careful observation—and the help of a local worker—we could make out peaks of smaller temples, as yet unexcavated. Thousands of undiscovered structures lay buried in the surrounding jungle thicket. Whoops of howler monkeys ricocheted through the air, and we were warned that jaguars and cougars roamed freely just beyond the cleared areas. Slinking breezes, available only this high above the ground, lent a mystical air to the site.

Julia followed my words intently, even as I stumbled over some of the descriptions. She nodded as I spoke, and I realized that I was making a semblance of sense, that I was somehow managing to tell a story in Spanish.

"It is my dream to visit Tikal," Julia said. "If my health and my immigration issues are ever solved, I plan to bring Vasco and Lucita to Tikal."

It should have sounded bittersweet, but it didn't. It should have been regretful, disillusioned, frustrated, furious. But it wasn't. It sounded hopeful. Hopeful! How on earth could Julia Barquero be hopeful?

"*¿Tiene esperanza?*" I asked incredulously, before I could catch myself. I was horrified to see myself so determined to ferret out what I knew to be the spiteful truth, but the question spat itself out.

"*Por supuesto,*" she replied, matter-of-factly. Of course. "*Tengo mucha esperanza.*"

I stared at this woman—exactly my own age. Our children were the same ages. We were in the same stage of life. But chance had thrown us on the opposite sides of the border and with the opposite genetics and there was nothing I could do about it. Her children were going to lose their mother—it was only a matter of time. How could she be hopeful?

I knew that her cardiologist was trying to get her on the transplant list, but the chances were infinitesimal. God, if only it were her kidney, not her heart. A kidney, at least, could be harvested from a cadaver, could even be donated by a living relative. But a heart usually required a healthy person to die of head trauma, and the window of harvesting opportunity was fleetingly small. I turned my gaze away; I couldn't look any longer. For whatever reason, Julia Barquero had hope. Even if I did not, the least I could do was let her enjoy the succor of her hope.

When Julia stood to leave, we stared at each other for a moment. Her eyes were dark and strong, and her gaze did not falter. Maybe it would indeed turn out all right. Maybe her steadfast *esperanza* wasn't crazy at all. She gave me a hug that was muscular, confident, and I allowed myself to relax into her embrace. I wanted to tell her how much I admired her, how I wished I could have as expansive a confidence in the world as she did. But for the moment there was something relieving about simply letting her energy take the lead.

⋙

The day went by quickly, filled with my patients who'd managed to get to the hospital by subway or on foot. The snowstorm, strangely enough, appeared to have a salutary effect on everyone. If you didn't have to dig out a car or shovel a driveway, snow was something that could be enjoyed. And in a city that had successfully concretized every square inch of a former deciduous forest, an invasion of the natural world was a felicitous interruption of normal life. Each patient seemed energized by the overriding cleanness and beauty of the city. Everybody had his or her own story to share about the snowstorm.

As I walked toward the front desk to get my twelfth chart, I spotted Mrs. Geng sitting in one of the exam rooms. She was with her home attendant, talking to our social worker. I wondered what she was doing here; she wasn't on my schedule for a medical appointment. I hoped there wasn't a problem.

I popped my head into the room. "Is everything okay?" I asked the social worker.

The social worker waved away my concern. "Mrs. Geng is just here about some paperwork," she said. "We need to reauthorize home services before they expire. I'll drop it off for your signature as soon as I'm done."

"How are you, Mrs. Geng?" I asked, entering the room more fully. The attendant was also an older Chinese woman and spoke a smidgen more English than Mrs. Geng. She was doing the translation for the social worker.

Mrs. Geng smiled and nodded. "Fine. Fine." She wore a gray boiled-wool coat and a Himalayan cap that was pulled low over her eyes. Two mufflers wound around her neck, and her feet were clad in sturdy worker boots. Her cheeks were flushed from the outdoors.

The social worker put down her pen in midsentence and turned toward me. "Did you know," she said, "that her husband went back to China for good?"

Mrs. Geng and the home attendant echoed her like a Greek chorus. "Husband in China," they repeated, nodding their heads somberly.

I let out a long sigh as a bitter flash of that uncomfortable day in their garden crept up on me. I still felt tarnished, as though I'd somehow abetted a crime. "Yes," I said regretfully. "He is indeed in China."

"Husband in China," Mrs. Geng and her attendant intoned again.

"I'd thought he was only going for a few months," the social worker said, her hands scalloping the air in wonder. Apparently, she'd only just now been informed of the reality.

I gazed at Mrs. Geng, bundled up against the vagaries of nature—an unexpected snowstorm in March. Was her soul equally fortified against the vagaries of human nature—an unexpected life chapter as a single elderly woman?

Part of me almost wished that her Alzheimer's disease would progress a little more, just enough to blunt her awareness of this pain. Then, in what felt like a direct reaction to that thought, a wave of fury toward Dr. Chan swept over me. He'd gotten out while the going was good. He'd exited stage right just before the hard part commenced, choosing a better life for himself at the expense of his wife. By leaving now, he was going to spare himself the misery of her descent into dementia.

Dr. Chan would be living the comfortable life in China while his wife would lose her ability to walk, to dress, to toilet, to feed herself. He'd be in the sunset of his retirement while his wife would forget where she lived, who her daughters were, how to speak. He wouldn't have to see her in a nursing home, in diapers, with oatmeal stains on her gown, with interns grimacing at the foul smell and questioning each other about why she was being kept alive.

I leaned back against the door frame, hating how this anger made me feel. The truth was, Dr. Chan could easily die before Mrs. Geng—whether he was east or west of the Pacific Ocean—and be absent for the dreadful demise to be wrought by Alzheimer's. He was more than fifteen years older than his wife and had diabetes and hypertension to contend with. His risk for vascular disease was prodigious. These months could be the last few of his life. Should he really be begrudged this final wish of returning home?

I shook my head to clear the thoughts; the whole issue was making me dyspeptic. I bade farewell to Mrs. Geng, knowing that I'd surely see her on our street when I was out walking Juliet. I was glad that I had a way of keeping close tabs on her.

I took my chart and continued back toward my office. Dr. Chan's wooden carving was still hanging from the bookshelf where I'd placed it eight months ago. Part of me was tempted to tear it down and dump it in the garbage. I was angry at Dr. Chan for being selfish, for abandoning his wife. But I could identify with his urge to grab what was important in life, and—I had to confess—part of me respected him for doing it and not writing it off as futile just because he was ninety-one years old. I hoped I'd have half as much moxie when I was that age. The carving stayed where it was. The red tail fluttered—as it always did—when I opened the door for my next patient.

—⊱∞⊰—

Samuel Nwanko was on the list for today, but I wasn't surprised
that he was the one patient who didn't make it. He lived almost
two hours from Bellevue, and I was glad he didn't attempt the
trip. In any case, we had moved away from the traditional doctor-
patient relationship. The SOT program had helped him find a retinal specialist at another hospital, and Samuel had started a series
of surgical procedures there. He really didn't have any other active
medical issues that would require continuing visits at our clinic.
We'd met a few times outside of the clinic as he shared his story
with me, knowing that I was writing this book.

Samuel didn't have much free time these days. He had finally
started school at a local community college and even managed to
land a part-time job in a nearby hospital, helping in the supply room.
I'd been so nervous contemplating his first day of classes and work.
I wondered how long the stares would last. Hopefully just a short
time. It would have to be, I told myself, that his classmates and
coworkers would be able to see beyond the superficial. After
a few days, they would get used to it. After a few weeks, they would
get to know the robust, unique person beyond the face. In a few
months, Samuel would blend into the environment, would be part
of the school and hospital world, and he'd finally be able to pick
up where he'd left off.

Recently he'd e-mailed me a flyer. The retreat where he was
living had hosted its annual New Year's fund-raiser. It was a
candlelight dinner, with a concert "featuring our own Samuel
Nwanko."

I was taken aback by the emotion this generated in me. It was
the way the retreat phrased it—"our own Samuel Nwanko"—that
brought the lump to my throat. This group's members had taken
Samuel in, considered him their own. The love and pride evinced
by that choice of wording was so palpable...and so relieving.
Somehow this one phrase assured me that Samuel would be okay,
that he'd find his way in the world.

I had no illusions, however, that it would be straightforward,
and his letter that accompanied the flyer reinforced that. *I have*

been thinking of giving up music, for personal reasons, he wrote. *This was probably my final concert.*

I knew how much music had been an integral part of his life, his very survival even, but obviously his relationship to music was more riddled with conflicting emotion than I could ever understand. Having had my own opportunity to weave music into the core of my life in the past few years, though, I could appreciate how agonizing would be the process of closing it down.

I imagined the final concert—Samuel sitting at a worn but serviceable Steinway, a roomful of candlelit tables around him, the faces of the audience flickering in and out of focus. The keys would be silky to the touch, with a give that was familiar and welcoming. But the music that emerged would be a thorny mix of beauty and pain. The stinging associations would be impossible to whittle away. Maybe while he was playing the last notes it dawned on him that the only way forward was to decisively cut away this tie to the past.

But in my heart of hearts, I hoped that this wasn't the case. I hoped that the difficult memories might eventually recede of their own accord, without snuffing out his music in the process. Perhaps he just needed a break, time away from the emotional intensity of music. Maybe after he had time to heal, he would find that his music was still waiting for him, still alive in his soul.

I could only hope.

⸺⊗⊗⊗⸺

When I left clinic at the end of the day, it was still light out, the telltale sign that spring was approaching. My backpack was loaded down with the journals I hadn't read, the mail I hadn't responded to, and the manuscripts I hadn't reviewed—things I'd toted to work hoping to finish and was now, yet again, toting back home. The snow hadn't ceased but its pace had lessened, lacy oversize flakes tripping lazily to the ground. Just enough to keep the snow white, to hold off—for the moment, at least—the inevitable conversion to the gunmetal gray of New York City winters.

I walked briskly past my apartment building and continued straight toward the playground, where I knew Benjy had taken the kids. The scene was undiluted joy. Naava was busy scooping handfuls of "snow cones" into her mouth until her lips were frozen. Noah was carving out an army of snow angels. Ariel was flying down the slide, over and over again, shrieking each time she sailed off onto the landing pad of snow. There was something so instinctive, so unfettered, about their affinity for the snow. Was it the whiteness? The coldness? The evanescence?

I recalled once reading about the "rapture of childhood," and as I watched my three children burrowing through the drifts, drinking in the physical freedom, this seemed to be it. They were just starting out on their own journeys, and I relished—and envied—their casual obliviousness to the process.

A snowball landed front and center on my jacket, immediately crumbling into powder since the snow wasn't wet enough for packing. Naava stood at the top of the jungle gym, with another lumpy snowball in her hand. She bit a mouthful out of it, then lobbed the remainder in my direction.

It would be dark soon. We should really gather the kids and get home, I thought. There was dinner, bath time, stories, and the rest to do. I knew that if we didn't get started soon everything would be delayed, and the kids would get to bed late, and it would be hard to get them up in the morning, and we would be late to school and late to work.

But the snow continued to flutter down on us, speckling our coats and hats with sprigs of white. The doggedness of the flakes amazed me—how could these weightless bits of fluff possibly succeed in besting this city of eight million? Yet they had. The unending concrete of New York City was now a peaceful tableau of white, even if it was just a temporary one.

I tossed my backpack to the wayside and dropped backward into the heap of snow. I sank serenely, deep into the downy drift. As the fine powder crested over my forehead and spilled onto my face, I realized that it wouldn't be so easy to get back up. But it was cozy, and it occurred to me that I could easily fall asleep here; it was sort of like the saggy hammock on our veranda in Costa Rica. Naava, Noah, and Ariel came gamboling over, toting armloads of snow to contribute to my indisposed condition. Dinner would just have to wait.

Acknowledgments

I am indebted to my patients who shared their stories and who took the time for extended discussions about their lives, their countries, and their families. Their perspectives on the world have widened my own. I have learned so much about politics, religion, illness, courage, and character, not to mention the occasional pointer on cuisine and past participles.

I want to thank Suzanne McConnell and Sandeep Jauhar for their insightful comments on the book. Reading an eighty-thousand-word manuscript—at short notice—is the mark of a true friend and sympathetic fellow writer.

Special thanks to Helene Atwan and the staff of Beacon Press for their steady support and encouragement. Helene has shepherded this project through its various incarnations with an unflagging confidence—and remarkably good humor—that has kept me inspired...and typing.

And it is Benjy Akman's patience, generosity, love, and sheer unflappability that make all of this possible. It's been a spectacular first decade, and I can't wait to see what will come in the second!